CHILDBIRTH CHOICES

IN MOTHERS' WORDS

Kim Selbert, M.F.C.C.

Mills & Sanderson, Publishers

1990

Published by Mills & Sanderson, Publishers

Box 665, Bedford, MA 01730

Copyright © 1990 Kim Selbert

Library of Congress Cataloging-in-Publication Data

Selbert, Kim, 1951-
    Childbirth choices in mothers' words / Kim Selbert
        p. cm.
    ISBN 0-938179-23-3 : $9.95
        1. Childbirth--United States. 2. Pregnant women--United States--Interviews.   I. Title.
RG651.S45   1990
616/4'0973--dc20   90-5959
                                                                                            CIP

Printed and manufactured by BookCrafters, Inc.
Cover design by Lyrl Ahern.
Photo of author by Joan Follendore.

Printed and Bound in the United States of America

This book is dedicated to my mother Royle Freund. For over thirty-nine years she has been a tremendous support in my life, and she's always there when I need her the most. I value her honesty and appreciation for life, her giving nature and invaluable guidance, and most of all, her love and friendship.

When I called her the day I found out I was pregnant, I remember she couldn't speak—she was crying and they were tears of joy. Mom, we've shared so many years of joy—memories I'll never forget. I will always hold on to them and because I'm a mother, I can pass them on to my daughter Adrienne. Thank you for giving me life and providing me with unconditional love—a treasure so few can say they were given. I feel lucky and also blessed by our friendship which has been enriched by our common bond as mother and daughter.

Acknowledgments

I'd first like to thank my agent and editor, Joan Follendore, for her professional guidance and personal enthusiasm. She believed in this book from its early conception in 1986, and has helped me to shape it into the book you now hold in your hands.

There are many people I'd like to thank for helping with the medical information. The biggest thank you goes to Laurence D. Colman, M.D., who shared his expert knowledge within a short span of time. He also provided me with an important interview. I also wish to acknowledge Nancy McNeese, C.N.M., Salee Berman, C.N.M., Victor Berman, M.D., and Norman Goldstein, for their medical expertise and assistance.

My caring and supportive husband, Roger Selbert, who doubled and trippled his efforts to do shopping, errands, driving, and foremost, being available for me with emotional support when I needed it the most. There couldn't be a more loving husband and father. Thank you, Roger.

I have also appreciated our live-in helper, Lauren Kelly. She has provided needed babysitting, cooking, and general help when I've had to work on the book.

I'd like to acknowledge the following people who gave me suggestions, read parts of the manuscript, or supported and nurtured me with their interest in the project: Arlene Arnold, Gail Howell, Elysa Markowitz, Rochelle Mayer, Gale Mynatt, Mary Pinkerson, Helen Reid, Deborah Rennie, Michael Rosenthal, M.D., and Loraine Stern, M.D.

Thanks to those who provided me with names of women to contact for interviews: Michelle Barone Bush, Gail Howell, Nancy McNeese, Deborah Rennie, and Sharon Seabrook. I also appreciate the offices allowing me to leave my flyers to pick up: L.A. Childbirth Center, Natural Childbirth Institute & Women's Health Center, and Women's Medical Group.

Of course this book would not exist without the women whose words fill the pages of *Childbirth Choices In Mothers' Words*. I am deeply grateful to all who wanted to share their stories with me. Their words are within this book.

Last, but certainly not least, my daughter, Adrienne Lee Selbert. This book would never have been written had I not given birth to her. I didn't know how much joy I'd have as a mother, but I know now what the many rewards are, and I appreciate my precious daughter, who has already given me so much. I'm looking forward to the future—to see her grow, to continue learning from her, and to treasure our relationship as mother and daughter.

Kim Selbert, 1990

Foreword

As a childbirth educator, I'm fond of telling my peers that I've learned just about everything I know about childbirth from laboring women. Of course there are the text and the journal articles that keep me busy for an hour or so every evening, and there is the information I learn from other childbirth professionals—childbirth educators, midwives, and physicians. But the stuff that shapes my books and my workshops comes primarily from the mother.

Today, I'm credited with having introduced the use of guided imagery to the childbearing public. But I'm not really responsible for that—laboring mothers are. They taught me what reduced the fear, the pain, the length of their labors. I simply follow their lead.

More than textbooks, even more than clinical training, the mother's experience is the best source of knowledge.

Anyone who helps women through labor, and anyone planning to have a baby, has much to learn from other parents' experience of birth.

That's why this book is so important. It is a collection of a wide variety of birth stories—what women chose and why they chose what they did.

Reading it will enable childbirth professionals to better understand how every labor, like every snowflake, is a unique event, and why options suitable for one mother may not meet another's personal needs. Reading it will give the mother a glimpse of the way others give birth so she can choose the best method for her.

Carl Jones, C.C.E.

Carl Jones is America's most widely read childbirth authority and the author of ten books, including the international bestseller, **Mind Over Labor.** *His methods for reducing fear and pain are taught in childbirth classes from Boston to Tokyo.*

CONTENTS

Part I
HOSPITAL BIRTH

Part II
CESAREAN BIRTH

Part III
BIRTH CENTER BIRTH

Part IV
HOME BIRTH

Part V
MULTIPLE BIRTHS

Introduction

Childbirth Choices In Mothers' Words is a collection of birth stories as told to me by each mother. As a Marriage, Family, Child Counselor (M.F.C.C.), specializing in pregnancy and childbirth, I help women prepare for their birthing experiences. I listen to fears, hopes, and dreams about their births, and ready them as realistically as possible for childbirth and parenting.

All the information herein is factual, with documentation on file in my office. The names are deliberately changed, unless the mother requested her name be used. Please do not attempt to use the procedure described without first consulting a qualified medical professional regarding your individual situation. The author accepts no responsibility for the use of these procedures.

Birth is a powerful event, and when it doesn't live up to your expectations, your self-worth and confidence can be damaged. As a new mother, it's important to feel adequate about your mothering, and when your self-image is less than optimum, it affects your attitude toward the baby, and the baby's response to you.

It's hard to pave the way for everything that may occur during birth. "Hope for the best; prepare for the worst" seems to be sound advice. A woman expecting her first baby should:

1. *Become as informed as possible about pregnancy, birth and parenting.*
2. *Trust those who will be assisting at the birth.*
3. *And let go of expectations for the perfect birth experience.*

Before I became a mother, the high expectations I created made it difficult for me to accept the birth that actually happened, and although I was a M.F.C.C., I had limited knowledge of, and no experience in, being pregnant and bearing a child.

It was a thrill to be expecting our first baby! We planned a normal delivery in an alternative birth center (ABC) room in a local hospital.

In my first prenatal exam, the doctor said, "You have a small pelvis so your chance of having a vaginal delivery is about fifty percent. It'll depend on the size of the baby, and how you progress with labor."

I considered the cesarean possibility, and when I came across books on the subject I glanced at them—even picked them up. Then I just as quickly put them back on the shelf, thinking, "I won't have a cesarean, so I don't need to read about them."

One of my nightmares at that time was giving birth by C-section. I recorded it in my journal:

> *"I was at a party when I was about six months pregnant. Suddenly my mother and sister drove me to the hospital. In bed there, people came to visit and asked me about the birth. I told them, 'I don't remember anything.' My mom said I had a cesarean and hypnosis was used to put me under. I lifted my gown and saw the scars—it looked awful. I cried in disappointment for not remembering the details of the birth, and for having had a cesarean."*

My fear of abdominal surgery included the element of being cut, but mostly I feared having no control over the procedure. At seven months along, the cesarean preparation class at our hospital showed us the procedure for a C-delivery. It didn't seem so horrible, but my husband Roger and I didn't think for a minute that would be *our* birth experience.

The baby's due date arrived. It was raining lightly and I thought, "This would be a perfect day to have our baby!" I went to my prenatal exercise class, the beauty shop, and a deli for lunch.

After a bowl of chicken soup, I went to my last prenatal exam and found I had toxemia—high blood pressure; a five-pound weight gain that week; protein in my urine; and swelling in my face, hands, and ankles. The doctor told me to go home and lie on my left side so the excess fluid in my body could drain. By lying on the left, there'd be less pressure on my bladder from the uterus, while the blood flow would increase—flushing out the toxins with the fluid.

That evening I went into labor, soon after the Dodgers won the World Series. I was glad about both things, but especially glad to know we'd soon have our baby. In the hospital, they gave me magnesium sulfate intravenously to control high blood pressure, and I continued to lie on my left side. Roger stayed, breathing along with me and massaging my back and stomach. His calm presence and words of encouragement were effective pain-killers against the tortuous contractions.

Everything seemed to be progressing, but at the end of twenty hours, after having become fully dilated and pushing for over two hours, the baby was stuck in the birth canal. Our doctor prescribed a cesarean, saying, "Even if you push for ten hours more, this baby won't be able to come out."

Roger and I agreed we'd worked hard, and now we had to go through what we never expected. I read the surgery consent form, and signed it. There was both relief and apprehension at the prospect of a C-section—I was exhausted from a long, hard labor, but I was frightened about surgery. I trusted my doctors would be skillful, and that my baby and I would survive with no problems.

Emotionally, the most difficult part was waiting over an hour for the only obstetrical operating room. It was very cold in there, and I shook uncontrollably until Roger helped me concentrate on breathing slowly, as we were taught in Lamaze. I started to relax when suddenly the pain during surgery caught me unaware as the baby was being removed from my vaginal canal. I moaned loudly through the oxygen mask, and the doctor said, "I'm sorry, I'm so sorry. Just a little longer and you'll have your baby."

There was incredible joy when the doctor announced we had a girl. We were gratified to hear her healthy cry. I'll always remember Roger holding our brand new daughter, and how beautiful she was.

Roger's face was wet with tears, and the pediatrician said, "How wonderful to see a father so moved by his child's birth." What he didn't realize (my sympathetic husband told me later) was that Roger cried for me. It hurt him to see me in such pain and be helpless to do anything about it.

Our doctors had given us every chance to achieve the birth we wanted. We were informed about each choice and decision along the way, and I'm thankful for the team of doctors and nurses we had.

The post-operative recovery was easy and uneventful, however the emotional recovery was long and painful. I felt sad for many months, and spent hours dwelling on the details—trying to understand what happened. I missed the exhilarating experience of mothers who deliver their babies vaginally and consciously. I was consumed with grief and disappointment when I talked with them, and they couldn't relate to my distress. So I buried feelings and cried alone. Before the birth, I kept my birth fears to myself. After the birth, I was afraid to express the intensity of emotions inside me.

After months of sadness, I joined mother-infant group discussions on infant development and adjusting to motherhood. I lasted but one session in the first group—they'd all had the birth experience I wanted, and I felt so sorry for myself [that] I sat silently crying.

In the next group, some women had actually chosen cesarean under questionable circumstances. I was able to share my story, and even see it wasn't the worst possible scenario. I learned it was all right to mourn the loss of the birth I expected.

Psychodrama training was a major turning point for me. Playing my mother, I reenacted my vaginal birth while another group member played me being separated from my mother's body. I realized it wasn't very different from a cesarean birth. In fact, my baby was kept near me and I was more aware of what was happening than my mom had been. My husband sat right next to me and held Adrienne immediately, showing me how lovely she was. My dad had been in the waiting room, and saw his baby girl through the nursery window, hours after I was born.

I read those books on C-sections—that I should have read while I was pregnant. Then I would have been prepared, known what to expect, and [I would] not [have] been so frightened and disappointed. But reading them after the fact still helped me understand, accept and appreciate C-sections.

A year after Adrienne was born, I created, as a therapist, a mother-infant group and a prenatal support group. Working again helped my self-esteem, too. I needed to do something I wanted to do away from the baby, and not be solely a mother.

I had faced my greatest fear when I gave birth to our daughter. It was an experience I'll never forget, and the one from which I've learned the most. It taught me to accept my fears, to face them and to move on with life.

Part of my healing process was a dream two years later:

"I was home alone, in light labor with my first child. I pushed and panted and eased her out. I felt powerful, in tune with my body and with the baby, relaxed, contented, elated and wide awake."

That dream may become a reality with my second birth, if I choose to have another child. The old adage is no longer true, "Once a cesarean, always a cesarean." Circumstances can change from birth to birth, and each birth is treated individually. Now there are many vaginal births after cesareans. But should you need a cesarean, be grateful they're available, and that your baby can be brought into this world by capable, loving hands. Having a cesarean is *still* having a baby, and having a healthy baby is more important than the type of birth you have. Having a baby is what it's all about!

There are many other possible problems in giving birth, and the most common ones are described here—by the mothers who experienced them.

This book is written to prepare you to "expect the unexpected."

Kim Selbert, M.F.C.C.

Part I

HOSPITAL BIRTH

Alternative Birth Center Room (ABC Room)

The alternative birth center (ABC) room was created in the late 1960s, as an alternative to the standard, separate labor, delivery, and recovery rooms. An ABC room is nothing more than a glorified labor room, often with flowered wallpaper, a double or queen-size bed, and a rocking chair. The room is devoid of medical equipment, since the hospital is trying to create a bedroom atmosphere for women who qualify as low-risk birth patients. Women aren't able to use the ABC room if they have hypertension, diabetes or toxemia. Some hospitals discourage use of the ABC room by women having their first baby.

Before checking-in to an available ABC room (most hospitals have one, some have two), the laboring woman gives a urine specimen and has her blood pressure checked. Also, a strip reading is taken with an external fetal heart monitor: two belts, holding two metal discs, are strapped around the woman's abdomen, and the discs pick up uterine contractions and the baby's heart rate, to record them on the monitor, over a twenty to thirty-minute period.

After this strip reading, if the baby's heart rate stays consistent, and the mother's blood pressure stays low, she can go into the ABC room, continue with labor, and eventually deliver her baby there. Friends and relatives may attend the birth, and the number accepted is determined by the hospital's protocol. If the mother has other children who want to be present during the birth, they are generally required to take a sibling preparation class at the hospital, and have adult supervision at the birth. This person should be someone other than the father or coach.

Advantages of the ABC room include: staying in one room for labor, delivery and postpartum; the flexibility of having children at the birth; a certain amount of privacy, since the couple is left alone more of the time; and the nearness of medical intervention if it becomes necessary (at that point, the family would have to leave the room).

Technical Reference: *Laurence D. Colman, M.D., specializing in Obstetrics, Gynecology, Infertility and Endocrinology, Santa Monica, California*

Rebecca

Rebecca had her third child in an alternative birth center room in a local hospital, with her husband and two older children in attendance. Her fourth child was almost born there, too. She compares and contrasts her four births, and discusses the advantages of having a family-centered experience.

I had my first two births at a large hospital, eleven-and-a-half and ten years ago. At that time, there were a zillion rules about how they did everything. You had to stay in bed, and have an IV, and all sorts of things. I was in the hospital about twelve hours with the first one. I had to be in bed, and it was very difficult.

With my second labor, I was in the hospital for a very short time before the birth. It seemed easier on me to stay home, and keep moving.

I wanted to be sure to have that situation for my third birth, and I discovered that an alternative birth center (ABC) room offered it. When our third child was born, Celina was five-and-a-half, and Jacob was seven, and I wanted them to be part of the experience. The main reasons I wanted to use the ABC room were: to include my children at the birth; to allow me to move around; and to do what I needed to do during labor and delivery, whether that meant taking showers, having massages, or whatever I wanted.

My water broke, about sixteen days before the due date, and it took a really long time for labor to set in. I didn't go to the hospital until I was in active labor—on the Fourth of July. There was no one around, so they let us stay without actually checking me in.

Jacob and Celina came in with an adult friend of ours who supervised them. It was great! The kids were comfortable and they got to watch the fireworks from the ABC room window. Soon after the show, Jacob fell asleep, while Celina continued to watch me in labor.

4

I was most comfortable pacing. And cold wash cloths, on the back of my neck, helped in the summer heat. When I became too hot, I took a shower, which was adjacent to the room. I'd shower off and cool down. Even though I didn't have back labor, the water beating on my back helped to take the edge off the pain for a little while. At some point, I couldn't stand to have the hospital gown on, so I took it off. It was just my family in the room, so it was fine with me to be naked. That's what I needed to do. Whatever I could do to get through it, I did.

I didn't have any medication, and I didn't even have an episiotomy, because the doctor massaged the perinium with oil. He learned this procedure from a midwife he knew. I had episiotomies with both my other births.

Unfortunately, the cord was wrapped tightly around baby Jesse's neck, so they couldn't get him to breathe properly in the room. The pediatrician had to whisk him into the nursery, which was literally next door. He was there immediately, and my husband, Lee, went with Jesse.

The doctor finished with the afterbirth, and made sure I didn't tear. Jacob and Celina climbed into bed with me. We just held onto each other. Our friend, Pat, who was watching the kids, stayed with us. She kept calm, and that helped me get through my concern about Jesse. I didn't want to fall apart in front of Jacob and Celina. They were disappointed because the baby couldn't be in the room with us, but Jesse had to be taken care of in the nursery.

The doctor, who was a family practitioner, went into the nursery as soon as he was done with me. He played messenger, coming in to tell us what procedures they were doing, and how Jesse was responding. I'd then explain it to the kids, as calmly as I could. The main thing was we were together, going through it as a family. Jesse had to stay in the incubator overnight, as a precautionary measure, but he was doing fine.

The kids went home, and I went into a regular room. Celina and Jacob still remember Jesse's birth as a positive experience, even with the problem. They were able to see that something could go wrong, but it was handled, and there was nothing further to worry about.

I didn't feel comfortable with the idea of a home birth. I was just enough aware of what the problems could be, and that also kept me away from a birth center. That would have been tempting fate. I wanted the flexibility of what home offered as a setting, but I wanted to be in a hospital "just in case." And we had that "just in case" with Jesse. Fortunately, it turned out to be nothing in the end, but it could have been something. I knew once you're actually delivering your body just takes over. I wanted the best of both worlds, and that's what I felt the ABC room offered.

There were qualitative differences between my third birth and my others. Going into labor this time was an easier transition from the end of the pregnancy. The other times, a sudden, different thing happened—I was in labor and having the baby. There were tubes and nurses and monitors. It didn't seem like a natural extension of what had been going on. Also, being moved into the delivery room from the labor room interrupted the flow. It was much smoother for everyone to stay in the ABC room for everything. All the things done in the first two births, with the monitors and tubes, increased my tension—especially during the first birth. Every time they went to check something, my anxiety level went way up. Had I been able to do it in a different setting, I would have felt better about it.

The first birth was pretty difficult because the labor pains were in my back almost the whole time. Then they picked up fetal distress and were going to do a cesarean—not an emergency one—but they took blood first, and moved me into the delivery room. Right before they were to prepare me for anesthesia, the doctor checked again to see if I had fully dilated, and I had.

The baby hadn't dropped into the lower part of my pelvis, but after having back labor for ten hours, when they told me to push, I pushed very hard. They never had to use the forceps they planned to, and he was delivered in twenty minutes. It was wild! I was in a cesarean delivery room, and there weren't any stirrups on the gurney. I asked a pediatric resident and a nurse to hold my legs. When they said, "Push," boy, did I push! And he was delivered without any problem. The umbilical cord was wrapped around his chest, but it wasn't dangerous, as with Jesse—having it around his neck.

My second child, Celina, had a very easy birth. I was in labor only six hours. We didn't get to the hospital until five-thirty, and she was born at six-oh-one. Even though her birth was easy, I didn't entertain the idea of having my third at home or in a birth center.

6

For my fourth birth, I started out in an ABC room, and had to be moved into the delivery room, because he began showing signs of fetal distress. They couldn't figure out why, and then he became stuck in the birth canal. They thought they were going to have to do a forceps delivery, so . . . they wheeled me into the delivery room. Once there, the kids couldn't come in with me.

Fortunately, the forceps didn't have to be used. I didn't even need the perineal massage, because he came so quickly. The kids knew the baby was born, and went to the nursery to see Ari, even before they came to see me. It was easier for them in Jesse's birth, because they weren't separated from me. They could stay right with me in the ABC room.

Another thing I did differently at Jesse's, was a method learned from Lamaze classes—to use a picture as a focal point—something I could look at while I had contractions—as a way to concentrate and relax during that time. Mostly, I walked around the ABC room during labor. That particular kind of discomfort makes me antsy. It's even true if I get the stomach flu. I can't stay still with that kind of pain, so I just kept moving—walking back and forth, back and forth.

It was really funny because I'd say, "Here it comes again," and little Celina looked around to see what was coming.

She'd say, "What's coming? I can't see anything."

Between contractions, I'd sit down. When I felt another one coming, I'd stand up and announce, "Here it comes again," and return to my pacing.

Our friend explained to Celina over and over again that it was the contraction, it was a feeling inside, and what I said was just an expression. She told her this is the way the baby would be able to come out.

What also helped me during labor was placing cold washcloths on the back of my neck. When it got too hot for me, I'd take a shower. Standing under the water helped by cooling me off . . . and helped to take the edge off the pain.

I was late delivering the first two pregnancies, so it was nice to have started labor early this time. My theory on why the third one came early is that doctors have found if you start to dehydrate, it can cause contractions to start. The week before Jesse was born, it was beastly hot, and I have a feeling I didn't compensate enough for how hot it was. I was drinking, but I may not have been taking in enough fluids. It was up in the nineties, even here in Santa Monica. There was no relief, so I have a feeling I became dehydrated.

Giving birth totally changed my notion of modesty—I don't think I have any, anymore! I follow the social conventions, but the idea of my body as this very private thing stopped, because that's not what it was. It's not that I feel detached from it—it's that I don't feel I'm as wrapped up in it, in terms of modesty. I still care about how I look, that hasn't changed. But when my body is taking over and doing the function that it's doing, it doesn't matter what kind of image I have of myself.

When I went for a gynecological exam or had a problem with my breast, and went to a breast man for tests, it didn't upset me. I could separate myself from my body, because my body is serving certain functions it needs to do. I think that's something I couldn't have done prior to having children. It's good, and makes it easier for me to be comfortable around my kids—for them to see me when I'm naked. This wonderful thing contains us and serves its functions in various ways, but my body is not who I am.

Jesse's birth was even more of a family experience than I hoped it would be. Sometimes I get these glorified images of "the family" doing something together, but this time the vision was fulfilled. It was the last delivery for our family practitioner, who could no longer afford to do deliveries because of the enormous malpractice insurance required. His wife was the person watching Jacob and Celina, and she had never before seen her husband deliver a baby. He had been with her when she had their children, but she had never seen him as a doctor delivering a baby. So it was a wonderful and special time, and we were all connected to each other at this birth. I know it made it easier, for our doctor's last delivery, to be with a family he has a personal relationship with, and to know he would see this child after the birth.

It was memorable for Jacob and Celina, too, because they saw their baby brother the first second he existed, the same way their dad and I did. The kids weren't separated from this event. The parents didn't go and have this baby, and then later the children were introduced to him. They could see immediately he was part of the family. They accepted him easily. Maybe because he came early, and had some problems, they felt protective of him and cared for him and about him more than if a strange baby had been brought home to them. I think it was less threatening, because they were concerned about him.

Jesse was born at eleven at night, and we went home the next afternoon. Jacob and Celina went home with the doctor to spend the night, and my husband Lee stayed with me in the hospital. When the doctor came to check on me in the morning, he brought the children with him. They stayed with me in my room, with Jesse there, until we all went home about two o'clock. I didn't want to stay in the hospital, away from my family. I settled myself on the couch in the center of everything, and stayed there with the baby for a couple days, until I was ready to be up and about.

I remember something fantastic that one of our Lamaze teachers told ... the husbands, "Keep reminding your wife she's going through this to have a baby." It's so easy to get caught up in what's going on in your body, you forget you're going to have this wonderful creature that you've really wanted. The birth ends up being very insignificant in the life with your child. However the birth turns out, it doesn't matter, as long as you end up with a healthy baby to begin this relationship. The birth experience recedes—it ends up being a good story that's interesting, but it doesn't hold a lot of significance beyond that.

The first time I was upset that it was going to be a cesarean birth. What scared me most was that they were going to put me under, and I was terrified of having general anesthesia. Even if that had been the case, and upsetting as it might have been at that moment, I now know it would have just become a story—no matter what kind of birth my child had. It's great fun to tell the children all the drama that went on at each of their births. They love hearing about them. But they're not really important, compared to the relationships.

Parents are so focused on the birth itself, because they can't picture life after that birth. It's good to remember you don't have much control over what's going to happen at birth. Something may happen that you're comfortable with, and then something may happen you don't expect—you don't really know what you're going to experience.

Lee was more comfortable with the third birth, perhaps because he'd been through it twice before, or because it wasn't like a hospital setting. He would walk with me, hold my hand, stretch out on the bed between contractions, and he also liked having the kids there. I'm not sure what factors made it work better, but he was definitely more comfortable and didn't feel as self-conscious.

The nurse wasn't in the room all the time—she came in and out, and was more relaxed than any nurse we'd ever met. She would say, "I'm available if you need me." And she'd tell us where she was going to be. When she came in, she explained what she was going to do before she did it, and asked me when it was a good moment for her to do whatever she needed to do. She was really terrific! In fact, she was supposed to go off-duty, but worked an hour longer, to stay until after the birth. She said she'd been through it all with us and wanted to stay until the end. Lee and I really appreciated that.

With this birth, there were no impediments to making me comfortable. Because of the way things went for our third child's birth, we planned another ABC room birth for our fourth child.

Introduction to Chapter 2
Breech Delivery

In the following story, a woman attempts a vaginal breech delivery, after reassurance by her doctor that a "frank presentation" is the safest kind of breech to deliver. With the advent of ultrasound diagnoses in obstetrical practices, doctors are informed of the baby's presentation well in advance of the due date. However, if her baby is in a breech position, an ultrasound scan should be repeated on the day the woman goes into labor, to verify that it's still breech. Many babies turn during the last few weeks before birth.

By the end of pregnancy, only four percent of all babies are in a breech presentation. The different types of breech presentations are: frank breech (buttocks first); single footling breech (one foot first); double footling breech (two feet first); knee presentation; and complete breech (knees are pulled toward chest, so both feet and buttocks are presenting).

Since many doctors are either unskilled at performing a breech delivery, or don't want to risk being sued if they attempt it and there are complications, they may suggest an attempt to turn the baby by version (gentle manipulation of the baby from the outside of the mother's abdomen) during the thirty-sixth or thirty-seventh week of pregnancy, rather than scheduling a cesarean section. Doctors found that when this procedure was done earlier than thirty-five weeks, there were two problems: if in doing the version, the baby became distressed and needed to be delivered, there were problems with prematurity; and even if the version was successful, there was still time for the baby to revert back to a breech position before the birth.

Currently, if a woman wants to attempt a version, she waits until her thirty-sixth or thirty-seventh week. The procedure is done in a hospital labor room, with the C-section room available to safeguard the small percentage who require an immediate cesarean. The woman is hooked up to an IV with terbutaline—the medication that relaxes the uterus. This drug accelerates the mother's heart rate, but it's not dangerous as long as it's monitored. It is the drug of choice, used when a woman goes into pre-term labor, to relax the uterus. The safe

11

use of terbutaline has not been definitely established. Its therapeutic benefits have to be weighed against any yet-undetermined harmful effects to the mother and child. This medication should be given only when your doctor determines it's absolutely necessary. Potential risks to mother and baby are: increase in heart rate; elevation of blood sugar level; and decrease in potassium level.

One or two doctors are present for the version. A diagnostic ultrasound machine is used to monitor the baby's position throughout the procedure. Once the terbutaline takes effect, the doctor's hands manipulate the fetus from outside the womb, through the mother's skin, to try to flip the baby forward or backward into a head-down position. There is some discomfort for the woman, but once the manipulations have ceased, the discomfort ends. After one or two attempts are made, it becomes apparent whether it's possible for the baby to be turned or not.

If this procedure necessitates an immediate C-section, the baby's chances of being healthy are excellent, because the baby is virtually full-term. Also, in most cases, the baby is turned into a head-down position, and so the woman has a greater chance of a vaginal delivery. Version is usually more successful on women who've had at least one prior pregnancy.

Technical Reference: *Laurence D. Colman, M.D., specializing in Obstetrics, Gynecology, Infertility and Endocrinology, Santa Monica, California*

Debra

Debra discusses her problems with infertility, and her first pregnancy. After two unsuccessful attempts at turning the baby by use of version, Debra has a vaginal frank breech delivery.

I had infertility problems for years—major surgery twice when I was twenty, and many different kinds of treatments. I even tried to get pregnant on my own and be a single parent. At thirty-two, I desperately wanted a baby, and started feeling like it wasn't ever going to happen—that I'd never get pregnant. I'd had a couple of false pregnancies—I wanted to be pregnant so badly that I had some symptoms of pregnancy.

When I least expected it, and when I let go of my obsession to have a baby, I became pregnant. I remember hugging the nurse when I got the results of the urine test. I couldn't believe it finally happened. I was really excited!

Because I had a history of endometriosis, which is an infertility disease, I had to undergo a pretty quick diagnostic ultrasound. It was done to confirm that it was a uterine pregnancy, and not a tubal pregnancy.

The next thing I had to deal with was the first trimester. For years, I suffered with migraine headaches. During the first trimester, with all the hormones changing, I had extremely bad migraines and had to be rushed to the emergency room on four of those occasions. I was treated with injections of Demerol, and even morphine at one point. I couldn't take my migraine medication any longer, so this was the prescribed treatment.

That was an awful experience, because I had a horrible fear that it was affecting the baby. During one of those emergency trips, before I was twelve or thirteen weeks pregnant, they could hear

13

her heartbeat. That helped reassure me that, even though they had given me injections to stop the pain, my baby was okay.

We moved into the second trimester, and the headaches subsided. Then I had sciatic nerve problems. I was ordered on bed rest for quite awhile. But I didn't care what I had to cope with, as long as I could carry the baby to term and know my child would be all right.

We had several diagnostic ultrasounds. In fact ... there was a group of doctors and student doctors who wanted to do an ultrasound scanning at no charge, as a demonstration, in the fifth month of my pregnancy. My boyfriend and I didn't want to know the sex of the baby prior to that. Then they started hinting around and said, "Sixty/forty girl." I wasn't really sure, because an ultrasound isn't always predictable.

I didn't have amniocentesis, and wouldn't have wanted it even if the doctor had recommended it. It had taken me so long to finally conceive that, even if there was a millionth-of-a-chance of miscarrying after the procedure, I wouldn't have risked it. If there was a birth defect, or something else to cope with, I would be more than willing, because I finally had this life inside of me, and I wanted this baby so much.

I remember [that] during my thirty-first week, I was having contractions and really panicked. Part of me thought, "Oh God, not now. Not after everything else. I can't have something go wrong." I went to the hospital and was monitored, and learned I had a urinary tract infection—not uncommon when a woman's pregnant, and this sometimes leads to pre-term labor. They treated me with an injection of terbutaline—a medication which relaxes the uterus—and the contractions stopped. To clear up the infection, I was on antibiotics for ten days.

The contractions started up again in my thirty-fourth or thirty-fifth week. I had three trips to the hospital with pre-term labor. During my thirty-fifth week, the doctor decided to try and turn the baby, since the week before they could tell she was in a breech position. They thought they should ... try the version the following week. During this procedure, the uterus is relaxed with medication and one or more doctors attempt to turn the baby from a breech position to a head-down, (vertex) position.

They did so many diagnostic ultrasounds to check her position. I probably had more ultrasounds than any woman I know. I think we had twelve or more. During the first version attempt, it didn't seem likely she would turn. That was a rough experience for me. The doctor doing the procedure didn't have a good bedside manner. I don't know whether she was overtired or what, but it wasn't pleasant. I was basically told, after being put through a great deal of pain in the attempt, that I had bought myself a C-section because I couldn't withstand any more pain.

My doctor, who hadn't attended me that night, was very upset I was given that kind of treatment. I was encouraged to try a second attempt with a doctor who had more experience in dealing with breech births and versions. This doctor was the first who told me, based on the size of my pelvic structure, that there was a good chance to deliver vaginally.

The second version attempt, which was done at thirty-seven weeks, wasn't successful either. The doctor used a lot more medication to relax my uterus. I was told I could have the C-section done that day, if we decided we wanted it. Otherwise, I was to schedule it no longer than one week away. They didn't want me to go past thirty-eight weeks, if I was scheduling a C-section, because they didn't want me to go into active labor. That could complicate the surgery, especially with the baby in a breech position.

I was very determined not to have a C-section. It wasn't so much being cut . . . I'd had a lot of abdominal surgery. To me, it was more an issue of really wanting to feel what it was like to experience labor and give birth.

The doctor told me it was a frank breech, and the only type of breech he'd attempt vaginally. Her feet were straight up like a "V," off to my left side. Her head was up on the right, and her buttocks were coming out first. There was no way she was going to turn after two attempts. She wanted to "moon" the world and all the doctors.

I chose to go into labor. Her due date was November 3, and I thought [that] with the premature contractions and all the other problems, she'd come early. As it turned out, she was ten days late.

I was miserable from the tremendous weight I put on. The doctor told me to gain about thirty-five pounds, since I weighed ninety-eight pounds before the pregnancy, and I'm five-two-and-a-half. I ended up gaining sixty-two pounds, so I was really uncomfortable.

I spoke with other women who had gained excessive weight in their pregnancies, and a lot of it was giving in to cravings, which I should have avoided. But I didn't think the extra weight was going to hurt the pregnancy—I even thought it might be better for the baby. My problem was more due to lack of exercise, because of the sciatica problems I had, and swollen ankles.

I tried to take little walks to get my labor going. Then I went to bed one night, and at four in the morning, when I rolled over, my water broke. No one can tell you what it's like to have that happen. You have to experience it. It gushed all over and thoroughly wet the bed.

I went to the hospital with my boyfriend, after calling the doctor. It was decided that, since I was attempting a breech delivery, they wanted to start me on Pitocin. I wasn't even dilated one centimeter. They also started it because my water had broken and they didn't want labor to go too long. The doctors were giving me every chance for a vaginal delivery.

An IV with Pitocin was started in my arm, and the contractions began quickly and intensely. I dilated rather fast. The C-section room was available, in case of a long labor or other complications. I was still determined to avoid one if I could. I'm a very stubborn person.

Once the Pitocin was started, I had to stay in bed. The doctor also wanted to give me an epidural at three or four centimeters. The problem was finding the anesthesiologist, who was at another birth. I was begging for demerol or something to take the edge off my pain. They gave me something that made me sick. I was in pretty active labor, and losing my concentration. My boyfriend was with me the entire time. We also had a good friend filming the whole thing.

I was dilating faster and faster, and the anesthesiologist was assisting at another birth. When she finally came, I was almost eight centimeters dilated. It was difficult to give me an epidural then, with such strong contractions. I had to lie so still, with contractions coming one on top of the other—it wasn't fun.

As labor progressed, they decided to place an internal monitor on her. There were so many doctors coming in on the case, because it was such an unusual delivery. There were student nurses who stayed on after their shifts ended to watch. By the time they moved me from the labor room to the delivery room, it had become very crowded in there. When I watched the film of the birth, I was amazed how many people actually attended.

My doctor placed the monitor, and a student doctor said, "You're going to put it on her buttocks?"

The reply was, "Generally it would be on the baby's head, but this will work just fine. We'll be able to monitor her in the same way." There was a little mark on her buttocks as a result of the internal monitor. After she was born, I used Neosporin on it, and it eventually went away.

I finally got the urge to push, while I was still in the labor room, and they allowed me to practice pushing. At nine-and-a-half centimeters, they decided it was time to move me into the delivery room. I remember, when they were rolling me in there, the orderly bumped the bed against the door and it jolted me.

Once in the delivery room, I heard the doctor say to me, "We're going to have to do a lot of things now, but they're things we have to do. So just work with us."

I kept on pushing and giving it all I had. I think they had increased the epidural so they could do an episiotomy.

An episiotomy is an incision made between the vagina and the anus, to make more room for a baby's head that is too large for the mother's opening, or when a quick delivery is necessary. The two types of episiotomy incisions are: a "medial lateral" which goes off to the side, at an angle from the vagina, downward; and a "lateral" which goes straight down from the vagina toward the anus.
Recovery time varies from woman to woman, although one or two weeks is generally needed. Sitting on a foam donut, and taking sitz baths can reduce the discomfort during healing.
—Laurence D. Colman, M.D., Santa Monica, California

Once, I reached down and felt her buttocks as she was on her way out. I finally gave my last push. Her buttocks came out, then her legs, and then her arms. Her whole body kind of dangled with her head still inside me.

Then they used forceps around her head, after a third-degree episiotomy was required. They pulled her head out pretty fast, clamped the cord, and asked Josh if he wanted to cut the cord. He did that and then, zoom! They had her on a table and were pumping oxygen over her head, helping her breathe.

After several minutes, she finally cried. Josh was a sobbing wreck, overwhelmed with emotion, by that time. She was fine, but until he heard her cry, he was very worried.

The doctor thought she wasn't going to be a large baby—another reason I was encouraged to attempt a vaginal delivery. But she was much larger than average—eight pounds, six ounces and only nineteen inches long. She was really plump, with a full head of brown hair and big blue eyes. We think they'll stay blue, even though Josh's eyes are brown and my eyes are green. His mother's eyes are blue ... so she'll probably keep the blue eyes.

They cleaned her up and then brought her to me. She cried after they got her lungs going, and kept crying. What was wild was, the minute they wrapped her up and handed her to me, she stopped crying. I wanted to be skin-to-skin with her, so they put the blanket over the two of us.

I held her for awhile, and then they took her to the nursery and put her in a warmer, because she was losing body heat. Josh carried her to the nursery, and our friend followed him with the camera to film the events that took place there.

They brought her to me awhile later and I nursed her. Giving birth was the most incredible experience. Even immediately afterward, as painful as it was, I said, "I would do this again." It was the most euphoric feeling in the world to see my baby looking at me. She was alert, and noticed people and everything around her.

They moved me fairly quickly from the delivery room to the recovery room. They did a really good job. The nurses and the doctors came around and congratulated me—amazed by the birth. It's rare for doctors to allow a woman to attempt a vaginal breech delivery. I was grateful she was so healthy. She had ten fingers and ten toes; everything was there. This was a miracle baby for me.

When I used to see other women who were pregnant, I'd be so envious. My heart would ache because I'd wonder if I'd ever be able to conceive. I thought my life would never feel complete if I didn't have a child and experience having a baby. It wasn't just giving birth. I wanted to feel every feeling of pregnancy, even the bad ones—to feel life moving inside of me and a baby kicking me. It's funny, but now I sometimes miss being pregnant.

I never expected to have the birth I ended up having. Not in a million years. I expected to have an easy birth, even though it was a first baby. My grandmother delivered one of her babies in the elevator going up to labor and delivery. She didn't even have labor pains; she had a headache. My aunt wasn't aware of labor except for having a backache. My mom's water broke, and I was born four hours later. Everyone had these easy births in my family, so I expected to have an easy one, too.

For whatever reason, Jessica turned out to be a pretty unique baby. There were a lot of people there. She must have wanted the attention. And she got it. Plenty of nurses and doctors were in both the labor and delivery rooms.

Giving birth helped me realize I'm a strong person. When you're really determined to make something happen, you have to believe in your dreams and not give up. It changed my whole life. I felt so bonded to this baby. When I first brought her home, I cried because I wanted to protect her from everything, forever.

What helped me most, when I was going through a long and painful labor, was the anticipation of knowing I would soon hold our baby in my arms. I'd finally see this little person who'd been kicking me all these months.

The bond of a woman with her child can be the most inspiring thing. That child will need you for quite awhile. I get so much from this baby, even now, when I'm giving to her all the time. I can run myself ragged, and I still have the patience of saints. Even when she was up every hour and wanted to nurse—in the beginning—I always thought, "She's a baby, and that's what she needs, and how she needs to communicate."

Donor Insemination

The following story discusses a single woman's pregnancy and childbirth experience. She decided to use donor insemination, and chose a sperm bank based on a recommendation from a friend. The sperm bank is not a health clinic, it merely collects the sperm from the donor and sells it to the recipient.

At her first appointment, she was shown three profiles of sperm donors to select from, after informing the director that her only requirement was to have a baby with blue eyes, like hers.

The director did some matching of the woman's hair and eye color, as well as her complexion, before selecting the specific donors. Photographs of the donors are available to the sperm bank staff for this purpose, but are not shown to clients, since the donors are confidential.

The profile of a donor, given to qualified applicants, lists the following information: physical characteristics, such as eye and hair colors; hair type; complexion; body type; height; ethnic, as well as racial group; ancestral origin, going back to donor's grandparents; year of his birth; educational history, including major and minor subjects; occupation; medical history of donor and donor's parents, including any illnesses or allergies present in the family; religious preference; blood type.

At least several profiles are provided, with the choice for additional ones upon request. The woman in the story suggests that when a woman is faced with having to select a donor, based on the profiles, she should go with her gut reaction.

Out of three profiles, she eliminated two, because in one case there was alcoholism in the family, and in the other the donor's parents were born the same year she was, and she thought that was like "robbing the cradle."

Once a donor is selected, the sperm bank arranges for the amount of sperm needed for the client. In this woman's case, she needed two vials a month, since there were going to be two inseminations each month.

Before the insemination takes place, the woman needs to take her temperature every day and note the changes. She uses an ovulation test kit to determine when ovulation (the release of an egg) is going to take place. If the kit shows the egg is about to be released, she picks up the reserved vial of sperm, which is packed in dry ice to keep it frozen, and takes it to her gynecologist's office for the insemination.

Some women take fertility drugs before the insemination process to stimulate the production of an egg, if that has been her problem. In this woman's case, she took clomid for five days before being inseminated, starting with the fifth day of her cycle.

The insemination procedure is very much like a pelvic exam. Before the procedure begins, a diagnostic ultrasound scan verifies that an egg is just about to be released. The sperm is also examined under a microscope to determine the motility and amount.

For the insemination, the woman lies on the examining table, as in a pelvic exam, with her feet placed in stirrups. The gynecologist inserts a speculum into her vagina, enabling the doctor to have a clearer view of the patient's reproductive organs. Then a needle-less syringe filled with the donor's sperm is inserted into either the fallopian tube or the uterus. Mild cramping occurs for about thirty seconds, but it's usually less painful than cramping during menstruation. The woman lies back on the table for five to ten minutes. Within two weeks, her gynecologist gives her a pregnancy test to see if the latest insemination was successful.

Technical Reference: *Laurence D. Colman, M.D., specializing in Obstetrics, Gynecology, Infertility, and Endocrinology, Santa Monica, California*

Toni

Toni, a forty-year-old single woman, chose to have a baby by donor insemination. She discusses her decision to be a single parent, the process of becoming pregnant, and the details of her daughter's birth.

The reason I chose to become a single mother was because "Mr. Right" had not come along. I had thought about it for five years when I started to hear my biological clock ticking ... I'd think about having a baby, and then I'd think of reasons why it would be too hard, and I'd forget about it. I was thirty-eight and I could hear the clock ticking much faster. I thought, "Gee, I'm probably not going to get married—at least no one is turning up right now."

Even though I didn't feel I was ready, I knew when I'd turn forty-five I'd be sorry. I didn't know how I knew that. I just had a sense there'd be something missing in my life at that point. There wasn't anything missing right now, and it wasn't that I always wanted to have a child. As a matter of fact, I really hadn't even thought about it.

I know a lot of women whose main goal in life is getting married and having babies. Those were never my goals. I just had a feeling that I'd be sorry, if at forty-five I didn't have a child.

I've had two careers in my life, and they didn't particularly give me satisfaction. I also found that at certain passages such as at the end of a decade, I'd get real itchy and want to do something different. When I turned thirty, I stopped teaching and went into business.

At about the time I was considering having a baby, I was thinking of starting my own business. I thought, "That's what I'm going to do in my forties." But as it turned out, what I wanted to do was be a mother.

23

The next five months I tried to get pregnant, with two inseminations each month. From November to March, I went through the ups and downs of the cycles. It was difficult to go through the ups and downs, because I've talked to other women who've been working on getting pregnant. It's the same thing—the emotion of test, test, test, test, test, ovulating, worry, worry, worry, get my period, depression, and then starting over again.

By the fifth month, I couldn't stand buying another test kit and peeing into the little cup every morning. And then I'd be waiting the two weeks with baited breath, to see if I was going to get my period or not.

When I think about it, for someone my age, I got pregnant pretty quickly. I know women who have tried a lot longer than I did. I was kind of frustrated at the end. After I'd have an insemination, I wouldn't drink, I'd be careful what I ate, and I wouldn't take any medication, not even Tylenol. I found myself really frustrated with that.

I was inseminated on March 9 and March 10, and I know I conceived on March 9. I was going to England for a week, about a week after the inseminations.

Once I knew I was pregnant, I immediately began taking very good care of myself. I also had many different kinds of tests, which are more recommended if you're over thirty-five. I had an ultrasound, an alpha feta protein test, and a chorionic villi sampling test which turned out to be my doctor's first CVS test on a patient.

I had a very experienced doctor doing the procedure. The only thing they cannot test for with CVS, that they can with amniocentesis, is the alpha feta protein test, which they can test with the amniotic fluid, and that's why I had the separate alpha feta protein test.

The CVS is like having a pelvic exam with many more people around, like Grand Central Station. There's ultrasound to place the fetus, and the doctor goes in through the cervix with a needle on a flexible cord. Some tissue is taken from where the placenta is going to form, and this procedure is done at nine weeks.

It took about five minutes, and there was less pain from cramping than during an insemination. The test results were available in two days, and it was wonderful! I found out all the chromosomes were present and in the right place, and that I was having a girl.

The hardest thing was not telling anybody once I had the information. I wanted a girl, and when I found out, there wasn't anyone to call. I think five people knew I was pregnant. I thought, "Oh, this is so great. I have such great news!" I had to call the sperm bank and my doctor's office to tell them.

I always wanted to know the sex of the child I was carrying. I wanted to bond that way—to have a name for this child. I really wanted a girl and spent two long days psyching myself into thinking I was having a boy, because the moment of truth was coming and I didn't want to be too disappointed.

I didn't want to announce I was pregnant until after the first trimester. I told my therapist, and she didn't even know I was trying to get pregnant. I told her the day I found out I was pregnant, and she said, "You're what? You didn't even discuss this with me."

And I said, "All the other times I've brought it up, it made me think why I shouldn't have a baby. Since I didn't bring it up to you, I just avoided questions like: 'How can I support a baby when I can barely support myself?' This time I thought, "Somehow I'll make do. I'll get by. If I worry about that, I'll never have a baby."

My mother brought it up to me about four years ago, that she really wanted to be a grandmother. There's just my sister and me, and neither one of us is married. My sister will probably never be a mother. My mother had said, "If you want to have a baby and you're not going to get married, I'm all for it." I didn't tell her about the pregnancy until after the first trimester. I didn't tell any of my friends.

One reason I didn't tell my friends about the pregnancy was [that] I wanted to get through the first trimester, rather than telling them and perhaps have the pregnancy end in a miscarriage. I didn't want to be in the "thinkers and tryers group," because I didn't want to go through the ups and downs with other women who were single and not sure they wanted to pursue the route of single parenting. I already knew I wanted to be a single mother.

I did have a scare in the twelfth week when I started spotting. My doctor didn't think it was a problem. Still, I was really scared. I had to tell my boss when this was happening, because I was scheduled to go to New York at that time. I couldn't see getting on a plane while this was taking place. I was so upset that it masked my excitement about being pregnant.

There was also the worry about how understanding people would be about donor insemination. I figured if I told them after the pregnancy was established and everything looked fine, I wouldn't have to go through any of the problems.

I went to see my mother over Memorial Day weekend, and I told her about the pregnancy. She went crazy and called everybody she knew. I was sure that would happen. Everyday she calls me and says, "How's my baby? How's my little grandbaby?"

To prepare for the birth, I took a series of Lamaze classes. I guess my way of dealing with things is not to worry about them too much and let them just happen. I had read the stories, and I had psyched myself up. I played a tape during the first three months that said, "This pregnancy's great; childbirth is going to be wonderful." I did stop listening to the tape, but in my mind I thought, "It's just going to happen, and I know people say how horrible it is but it'll be what it's going to be."

Then I went to Lamaze classes, and the instructor talked about all the awful things that could happen. Every week I'd come home and be upset. During every class, she'd talk about everything that could go wrong. The first week, she discussed all the complications during labor and delivery, like the placenta separating, and if your water breaks and there's meconium in it. Then she'd go into the details of each stage of labor and paint the blackest picture it could be. After that I thought, "I don't want to have this baby."

I remember thinking that a C-section would be better than the way she was describing labor. But then she'd talk about what a cesarean would be like, and I decided I didn't want any kind of birth. It turned out my labor was worse than anything she described. Now, when I think back on it after two-and-a-half months, I could probably do it again. Not that I *want* to do it again, but I could probably live through it again.

I asked my sister to be my support person, even though she's erratic and has been so in the past. She came with me to the class every week. She was so excited about this baby, and she's a very devoted aunt. As a matter of fact, my baby arrived the morning before the last Lamaze class, and my sister took the pictures to the class to show everyone. She was so supportive of me. My mother and sister were with me during labor and delivery.

I felt too old to be into natural childbirth. I remember sitting with my doctor the week before I delivered and saying, "I want an epidural. Be sure to give me an epidural." I knew I was going to get one, and the hospital said I'd have to be six centimeters dilated before I'd be able to have the anesthesia.

I remember my doctor coming in during labor and telling me she'd give me an epidural at two centimeters. She told me she couldn't give me the epidural when I'd first felt labor pains. That was really wonderful, because at that point I had been in labor for three hours and hadn't dilated. My contractions were now a minute apart and I dilated to one. I thought, "Well, if I can make it through another hour, I'll probably get an epidural."

After that it was wonderful! If I hadn't been able to have an epidural, I think I would have died! The epidural gave me instant relaxation, and it seemed to take effect in about ten seconds. I could talk, and I felt so comfortable. It took away all the pain.

The way things happened just before birth was strange. I was at the doctor's office nine days before my due-date. I had my regular exam and she said my cervix was about sixty percent effaced, which was the same amount as it was the previous week. The baby was really low, but she told me I had not dilated. She said, "I don't think you need to worry. Thanksgiving's coming. Just come back next week." I specifically asked if she thought the baby was going to come this week. She said, "No, I don't think so."

I left her office at three-thirty—arriving home about four o'clock. I spent the next two hours trying to figure out what was happening ... I knew I couldn't be in labor because I wasn't dilating. I felt kind of bad, with back spasms, and I figured out later I was having back labor. It took two hours for me to realize I was in labor.

I went from nothing, to contractions five minutes apart. Then, I left for the hospital after two hours of this, and the contractions became three minutes apart. By the time I was at the hospital, they were one minute apart. So, forget breathing; forget the textbook. The doctor was there and I said, "What is going on here?"

She checked me and said I wasn't dilating yet, but I was having contractions a minute apart.

Suddenly, I started to dilate. I went really quickly after that. From eight to nine o'clock, my contractions got a little more irregular—about two minutes apart. I dilated to two, and they gave me the epidural.

From nine to ten, I didn't dilate any further, and I thought I was going to be at the hospital all night. And then from ten to midnight I completely dilated. At midnight, I said to the nurse, "I know I shouldn't feel like pushing yet, but I really feel like pushing." She checked me and said it was time to push.

I remember looking at the clock and at the television—the "Tonight Show" was on. I wanted a Sagittarius baby, but right then it was Scorpio. After midnight, the sign changed to Sagittarius. Once the clock was at midnight, I thought, "Oh great, I'm going to have a Sagittarius baby." I was pushing, and I thought it was going to be a snap because her head was so low.

We went into the delivery room and I pushed and pushed for an hour-and-a-half, and nothing happened. I kept saying, "Isn't she moving? What's going on here?" She had a large head, and when I'd push she'd get close to the pelvic bone, but when I stopped pushing she'd go back in.

I remember they said, "Oh look, she has all this blonde hair." And I thought, "Great, she's right there." But after an-hour-and-a-half, still all they could see was the top of her head. She just couldn't get past my pelvic bone. Finally they said, "I think we're going to use forceps here." The use of forceps was the one thing they hadn't talked about in the Lamaze classes.

At one point I was lying on the delivery table and looking in the mirror at that absolutely unattractive angle, and said, "What am I doing here? What have I done." I think the realization hit me that I was taking on this tremendous responsibility—I was really going to have a baby! When they said "Forceps," I wanted to bolt from the delivery room. I had this vision of a Victorian doctor with a tall black hat, holding these big metal things. It was only because I trusted my doctor that I let go of my fear. I thought, "Let's go ahead and do it."

They continued the epidural anesthesia, and I had a local anesthetic for the deep episiotomy required. At the end of the third push, once they decided to use forceps, they held onto her head and she was out after two more pushes. I was worried about her skull being crushed. She had a little forceps mark, but didn't seem to be the worse for wear. She had a bruise across her forehead from banging into my pelvis for nearly two hours.

My sister held my hand and supported me as I pushed through the whole thing. My mother was somewhere in the background. She wasn't really sure she wanted to be in the delivery room. It was pretty daring for her. But she was there, and my sister and mother sort of snatched the baby away from me and fussed over her while the doctor did the repair work. I didn't notice the afterbirth—I just noticed the doctor sewing me for a very long time. She later told me it took time because of the forceps delivery.

As soon as they pulled the baby out they put her in my arms, and she was covered with vernix and some blood from the episotomy. I had her for about two seconds, and then the nurses took her away. They cleaned her up and did whatever they had to do.

Then I said, "Where's my baby? I can hear her crying." Finally, they brought her back to me from the nursery, and I held her. I was upset when they took her away from me. I guess they wanted to wipe the blood off her.

It's interesting what I remember. I got blood on my hand from her—it ran down my fingers. They didn't clean me up—I was like that the next day. In the wee hours of the following morning, I woke up and noticed I still had blood on my hands. It was like they didn't care about me.

I know when I first saw her I was glad she had red-blonde hair and looked like me, even though I was prepared to have a baby that didn't resemble me. I had this disbelief, and I still have it, in terms of knowing I produced this baby. I was really happy!

I didn't have any sleep, because she came at two-twenty-two in the morning on eleven-twenty-two. By the time I got to my room, it was about four o'clock. They pressed hard on the top of my uterus and did all the postpartum things they had to do.

I wanted to go to sleep, and I finally did around five o'clock. They woke me at six when they brought her to me. I only slept that one hour, and then I was calling everyone and telling them, "She's here—this little precious thing." She weighed seven pounds, fourteen ounces, and was twenty-one inches long.

I was really pleased she was so pretty. More than anything, she was exceptional looking. She was the only baby that had reddish-blonde hair, and she had lots of it—and it curled. Even though she had the bruise across her forehead, she didn't look like all the other babies—she looked different. I kept thinking, "Maybe that's because she's mine," but other people were saying how beautiful she was.

She didn't want to nurse at first. I thought something was wrong with her because she wouldn't breast-feed. She didn't want to eat for a couple of days. Then, after that, it turned out she just didn't want to eat from my breast.

When it was time to go home from the hospital, I was a little depressed because I didn't think I was ready to take care of this little creature all by myself. I thought, "What am I doing? I'm not old enough. I don't know anything about a baby!" My mother came and stayed with me. We battled over how I was going to do things. She told me how things were done when I was a baby, and [how] those things worked well then.

After I brought Sarah home, she had jaundice. A visiting nurse brought bili lights to clear up the baby's jaundice, rather than taking her back to the hospital for the same treatment I could provide at home.

When a baby has jaundice, it means there's a higher than necessary level of bilirubin [a by-product of hemoglobin] in the blood. The fetus requires a high level of bilirubin in order to obtain sufficient oxygen from the placenta, but after the baby is born, she doesn't need the same level because there is now air to breathe. If the liver doesn't break down enough of the bilirubin, the use of bili lights will. The baby is usually placed under the lights for six hours at a time, and then off for six hours, until the bilirubin is reduced to a normal level.
—**Laurence D. Colman, M.D.**, Santa Monica, California.

I continued to have problems with breast-feeding, yet I was determined to succeed. The nurses had shown me how to pump my breasts, and I continued to do that at home, so I could at least have the breast milk for her. When she started losing weight, they told me what to do. My mother told me to just give her a bottle and feed her. That's what I ended up doing, but I had to come to it on my own.

Being pregnant and giving birth was an experience I never thought I would miss, but having gone through it, I realize that it was important in terms of defining myself as a woman. It's like an initiation to womanhood. I've waited this long, and it made me more complete.

I don't look at it as an act of bravery. I had a baby because that's what I wanted. Everyone says I'm brave to have gone through all of this. My friends don't have any children—I'm the only person among my friends who has a child. I started thinking, "Well maybe I am brave, or foolish—one or the other."

I joined a support group of single women and mothers. I waited until after I was pregnant, because I didn't want to agonize over getting pregnant, and having all the doubts come out. I had one friend I could talk to about single parenting, and I'd bounce things off her.

At present, I find myself drawn to the women who are deciding whether to become single mothers or not. Maybe that's because I looked around the room and wondered how many women went through it the way I did. There really weren't any. There are women like myself who use donor insemination, but most women know the father. . . . Some of the women decide to adopt if they have problems getting pregnant, or they waited too long to begin trying to get pregnant.

I keep thinking I could have been more informed about what I was doing. I could have looked at all the sperm banks. It all worked out perfectly for me. I could have been much more cerebral about it. I know women who read every book there was, pondered all the possibilities. I just sort of fell into it, and I was lucky the sperm bank recommended a wonderful doctor. I had an easy pregnancy, and when I look back on the birth, compared to other women's stories, it wasn't that terrible. And I have this beautiful baby.

What I tell other single women who are thinking about having a baby is, "There is no right time. If you sit there and worry about how much money you make, how you're going to be able to raise a baby alone, you're never going to do it. If you want to be a mother, you really need to do it."

If I . . . [could] change something, I would have started earlier. It was lucky I got pregnant in five months. I meet a lot of women who are forty-two or forty-four, and they're starting to feel the effects of menopause, and still can't make up their minds. For me, it was looking at where I wanted to be at forty-five. I wanted to be a mother.

33

It was important for my doctor and her staff to be a strong support system for me. It felt like this was their baby, too. The doctor came in the night Sarah was born, and sat down with her and held her for about a half-hour and rocked her. She was like the father who helped give birth to her.

At least to my face, few people ever question me about who the father is. One friend asked me about the pregnancy, and that's because she was thinking about getting pregnant on her own and she didn't have the courage to do it. Everyone was very supportive.

I didn't broadcast to the world that it was donor insemination, but my mother did. And everyone was fine about it. They'd say, "Oh great, what is the father like?" They didn't seem to be too concerned about it. It was important that she was my baby. There was not going to be a father around, unless I met someone in the future.

There are so many fathers who don't take an active role. They walk out on their wives when she's pregnant. I have a cousin whose husband was killed in a freak accident when their daughter was three years old. She has raised that child by herself.

There are plenty of times when there isn't a father around. I had a father around who was not a good influence on my life. It's easy for me to say that it's better not to have a father, than to have a father whom you have to go through years of therapy for because of the problems you have as a result of inadequate parenting. That was my rationale. There are also fathers who just don't take an interest in their children.

I worry that there aren't any men in my life, like close friends or brothers. I don't have any male relatives who live close-by. She won't have a lot of male influence, but I don't know if that's good or bad. I'll just have to see what develops.

I have no idea what the father looks like, although I have his characteristics. There's no need to have a picture of the father of my child. I think that made me feel like donor insemination was a good thing. At least I wasn't picking someone just to use them. Certainly you don't know any more about a casual relationship than you do about the history of the donor you choose, and sometimes you know more about the donor.

When my daughter is old enough to understand, I'm just going to tell her she was really wanted. The important part was I wanted her and there was a means to have her.

I think a tough thing for me was what to put on the birth certificate next to "Father." That was probably the hardest decision I had to make. I wrote, "Declined to state," as opposed to "Unknown." I worried about that for a long, long time. I thought about what she'd use her birth certificate for, and what people would think.

She'll know about that before she needs to use the birth certificate for anything. I sometimes think about the idea of having a child when you're not married, and how the child has been referred to as illegitimate. I don't like that term at all. She's not illegitimate because she's mine. There are many unmarried women where I work who are having babies at a younger age than I did. To me, this wasn't an accident, it was a choice I made. And I'm so happy I made that decision.

Introduction to Chapter 4
Forceps Delivery

*Forceps were first introduced in England through midwifery prac-
tice in the seventeenth century, by the Chamberlen family. They were
designed to cradle the baby's head in a rigid metal frame, so the baby
could be pulled out of the pelvis without compression on the head.*

*There are a variety of forceps, ranging from small light ones
(designed to lift out the baby when it is on the floor of the pelvis), to
long flat ones (to help rotate the baby's head into the best position, the
occiput anterior position—with face to mother's back—for delivery).*

*Forceps are most frequently used when the baby's head will not
move down the birth canal, despite strong pushing on the mother's
part. They are also used when the latter stage of labor needs to be
shortened, for instance, if the mother has high blood pressure or there
are signs of fetal distress.*

*Certain conditions need to exist before forceps are used. The baby
is generally in a head-down position, although forceps can be used for
a breech delivery if the head is at or below the ischial spines (the
lowermost skeletal part of the pelvis). And the medical staff waits
until full dilation of the cervix occurs before making the decision to
use forceps.*

*When forceps are about to be used, the woman is placed in a
lithotomy position—legs bent, held up and open by resting the feet in
stirrups on poles fixed to the bed. A local anesthetic injection is given,
unless the woman has already had epidural anesthesia. Once the area
is completely anesthetized, the bladder is emptied by use of a catheter
and an episiotomy may be required.*

*The average forceps delivery takes between three and five minutes.
Marks may be left from the blades on the sides of the baby's face, but
these fade and disappear after a day or two. Forceps deliveries are not
dangerous at the present time, since the practice of **high forceps delivery**
(using a forceps with longer blades, which resulted in brain-damaged
babies in the forties and fifties) has been abandoned.*

*Doctors who have been adequately trained in the use of forceps
are at a decided advantage over newer trained doctors who are relying
more on the vacuum extractor. There are instances when a skilled*

doctor with forceps can assist a baby in a vaginal birth that would otherwise require a cesarean section. The forceps imitate the hands and should be used as such—to cradle the baby's head to help facilitate rotation into a better position for delivery.

Technical Reference: *Laurence D. Colman, M.D., specializing in Obstetrics, Gynecology, Infertility, and Endocrinology, Santa Monica, California*

Rita

Rita and her husband planned their first child's birth, with as little intervention as possible, at a local community hospital. It was a longer labor than anticipated, and then an unexpected forceps delivery was required. She was affected positively by her support team, which helped her through a difficult separation from her baby immediately after birth.

We tried for four or five months to get pregnant, although I stopped using birth control for eighteen months. That makes a difference too, because he, more than I, was nervous about having a baby. I think he wasn't sure he wanted to change his life that much. The longer we were married, the more we considered making this change. It made a big difference in his outlook, once we knew we wanted to add a baby to our relationship.

Over and over again, people told me, "Having a baby changes your whole life." Time spent with your baby is rewarding, but you don't have as much time for yourself anymore. You really have to be ready, because it's a big commitment.

I thought I was doing the right things by eating well and taking good care of myself—not drinking or smoking, not taking aspirin or any medication. Now, I would be even more conscientious before I'd get pregnant again. I'd learn more about pregnancy and nutrition. I didn't have an ultrasound scan the first time, but the next time I'm pregnant, I want one. I'd have been reassured if I could have seen the baby, and known everything was in working order. I'll do that in the future for my own well-being and peace of mind.

We intended to have a completely natural birth, if possible. That meant no drugs ... our doctor was really great and willing to go with the flow.

Almost twenty-four hours after my *back labor* pain started (all the labor pains were in my back, rather than felt in my abdomen area), and I was eight centimeters dilated, I had an epidural, which stopped my labor. I rested for about two hours, and began feeling some pain as labor built up again. At that point, my doctor arrived. He said he thought I'd have at least three more hours, and I wasn't sure I could take the back pain. I had very little contraction pain, but my lower back felt like it was going to break.

I moved a lot during labor; mostly from side to side. At one point I walked around, but then they placed an internal monitor on (me) and there was no getting up after that. They had to insert a metal probe into the baby's scalp, which gave a more accurate reading on the monitor. I could only move on one side or the other. I could sit up a little bit, but it wasn't ... comfortable.

My husband was with me the whole time. John helped by pressing on my back as hard as possible during contractions. He exerted so much pressure that *he* was sore the next day. The pressing on my back did help, but I was still feeling a lot of pain there. John was much better at coaching me with breathing than I anticipated, and that helped distract me from some of the pain.

My sister and mother-in-law were there for the birth. They both asked to be there, and I was hesitant. Before I got pregnant I said, "Oh, no problem." My mother-in-law had five children and was never awake during labor. My sister had been at another birth of a friend of ours, and said it was a wonderful experience for her. I didn't know if I wanted an audience or whether I wanted it to be private. Once I went into labor, it didn't matter. I thought, "Who cares? If it means that much to them, then it's okay."

What stood out about my labor was that I felt the pain all in my back. I figure that I was in labor when I was having the backache. It seemed to be happening at regular intervals, so then I knew that was labor. Other than the back pain, everything was fine. I don't have any strong complaints about it. My back pains started around nine o'clock in the evening, and I didn't go into the hospital until around three the next afternoon. At that point, I decided I was ready—my contractions were about five minutes apart. A great nurse met me. [She] was just going off her shift, but she helped me feel confident about how I was handling the pain.

The next nurse who came on was horrible! I wish I'd have found a way to get rid of her. Since it was my first experience and I was having back labor, and not really knowing what to expect, I didn't think to say I wanted somebody else. She was there about forty-five minutes before she finally asked, "Hi, how are you doing?"

I said, "Fine, except my back is killing me."

"Well, I think you better have an epidural right now. We're going to place a monitor on, and I really think you should have an anesthetic," she said.

I knew a monitor meant an internal monitor, which would mean I'd have to stay in bed and be more limited in movement. Also, an epidural might slow down the contractions.

I said, "No, I'm not interested in that, at least not at this point."

From then on, when she came in she'd encourage me to have an epidural or pain medication. She kind of took over as far as things went. When she actually did attach the internal monitor, some hours later, my water broke and I didn't know what was happening.

I asked her if my water had broken, and she said, "Well, no, I don't think so," as the whole bed became flooded.

Thank God I stayed in labor past her shift, because my next nurses were wonderful! It was eleven o'clock in the evening by then.

I was anxious and excited when I went into labor. I thought, "Now I'm going to know if the baby is okay." I didn't worry too much about labor. I figured, "I'll live through it; everybody these days lives through it. It's going to be hard, but I'll be able to do it." I didn't have any strong fears that I wouldn't make it. I was more worried about the baby—whether the baby was healthy, normal, all the things expectant mothers worry about.

When my labor stopped for two hours, they gave me an IV with Pitocin (an artificial hormone which increases the uterine contractions) to reactivate labor. The two-hour break was nice, because it was a relief for me. It was the first time in over twenty hours I could rest, and it was needed. When my backache started, I was really uncomfortable. I woke up the night before thinking, "This is just not right," but I could stand it. Once I got farther into labor, the pains became more intense.

41

My doctor said, "You just can't stop here," and they began Pitocin. That started the contractions a little. They told me I'd have to wait until the epidural wore off, in order for me to begin to push. I think it took a couple of hours of using the Pitocin before I started active labor again.

I pushed about two hours, but it seemed like fifteen minutes. I started out in the alternative birth center room, and then they moved me to a regular labor room, once I needed the internal monitor. Pushing was more work—a different kind of work. It seemed like my back was going to break during the longest contractions. Pushing was hard work, but I got excited doing it and it was rewarding.

During that phase, my nurses were wonderful. They knew exactly what to do and what to say to relax me. I sat up while I pushed. I had a birthing bed, but I don't think we ever dropped the lower part. I laid down between contractions, to rest and gather my strength.

The doctor told me, "The baby's big and he's in a posterior position." That meant the baby's spine was against mine. No wonder I had so much back pain! It seemed like he made a split-second decision about using the forceps, because I don't remember being given any anesthetic. Perhaps it was taking longer to push than he thought it should. Maybe he was fearful for the baby, I don't know. But he just went in and used the forceps at that moment. It really surprised me, because he said, "I think I'm going to have to help the baby," and that's when he used the forceps.

At one point, he said, "If you're not going to deliver in a couple of hours, we're going to have to give you a C-section." I knew I didn't want one, and told my husband, "No, I know I can do it. If it becomes a matter of safety for the baby, then okay.... Let's try not to do it."

My doctor said, "Okay, we'll keep going."

About two weeks before the due date, my mucous plug came out. I called my doctor to tell him and he said, "It doesn't mean a day, it doesn't mean a month." Before I called him, I read about it in a book, *Pregnancy And Childbirth*, by Tracy Hotchner, which I referred to throughout my pregnancy.

The mucous plug, also called "bloody show," seals off the cervix from the vagina to protect from infection. It is usually

*released when labor begins, but it can come out up to one
week before labor starts.*

Early in my pregnancy, I gained about three pounds a month.
Then one month I gained ten pounds. The doctor thought it was a
little unusual and he ran a diabetes test. Of course I panicked—I
thought, "Oh, my God!"

I went home and looked it up in my book. I wanted to know
how diabetes affects pregnancy. What I found out was, "Pregnancy
causes an increase in normal insulin requirements, which can lead
to increased maternal and fetal glucose levels, which in turn lead
to excessive fetal growth." I had asked the doctor too, but after I
left the doctor's office I always had more questions, and then I
could find some answers by reading in ... *Pregnancy And Childbirth.*

We had a great Lamaze teacher who gave us some booklets
she prepared for the course. I also got a lot of information from
them. They covered everything from nutrition to circumcision. It
discussed all the questions we had during the latter part of pregnancy, and all the big decisions we had to make.

I don't think I would have done anything differently, but because of what happened to my son, I'll be a lot more nervous the
next time, a lot more anxious about the baby. I think, until you've
gone through it and seen how beautiful a new baby is when it's
born, you aren't aware of how many things can go wrong.

The first thing I did when he came out, after the doctor said he
was a boy ... [was to have] my husband count his fingers and his
toes. I wanted to make sure everything was there. I looked at my
husband, and he nodded to reassure me everything was okay.

I was able to hold him, but not for very long because they felt
he was cold. Now I want to know why he was cold. Was he not
getting enough oxygen toward the end of labor? He did come out
purple. They wrapped him up right away and put him under warm
lamps. Everyone left as soon as they took the baby away. My
husband, sister, and mother-in-law left with the baby.

I was talking to the anesthesiologist who was still there with
me, and I asked, "Where is everybody?"

He said, "They went with the baby."

And I said, "Well, what about me?" At that point, I didn't
realize anything might be wrong, because they said they needed to
warm the baby up, and that's why they were taking him to the

nursery. They took cultures to see if there was a virus, and everything came out negative. They did a spinal tap to see if he had meningitis.... When they gave me a list of things it might be, they said he might have picked up some bacteria at birth.

After my son was born, he had a high white blood count. They took him immediately after the delivery. The pediatrician thought something might be amiss, so he kept Johnny in the hospital for five days. They put him on antibiotics and gave him all kinds of tests. They took all kinds of cultures; they did a spinal tap. I was there when they did his spinal tap, which was rough. Those things are with me a lot more than the birth. That's why I'll be more anxious the next time I have a baby.

Even though my baby was with me a lot, I wanted to go home, and I wanted him to come home with me. I was angry and wanted to know why they insisted on keeping him. They couldn't find anything wrong with him, but they didn't want him to go home until he was off the antibiotics. I was so emotionally involved, and I wanted my baby. I didn't want to go home without him. Originally I was going to stay one day, and I stayed four. I felt more depressed sitting in the hospital. He was still under observation in the nursery. I figured it wouldn't hurt for me to go home for one day. I nursed him for every feeding except the one in the middle of the night. I was trying to get my milk going.

For the type of birth and labor I had, I was somewhat prepared. In our Lamaze classes, the teacher went over back labor and we learned what it was and what we could do for it. I think it's important not to assume everything's just going to be the way you imagine it. It's important to be prepared for all aspects of birth, including cesarean. I remember even when the word cesarean came up in my reading, I said, "It's not going to be me."

When we were in Lamaze class, and the teacher talked about the possibility of cesarean, all the women looked around as if trying to figure out who might have that experience. None of us wanted to, and we all thought, "It's not going to be me." She was very thorough in terms of telling us what kinds of drugs or medications were available, and what the possible side-effects were on us and on the baby. I think I was well-informed about what to expect, although it's never what you anticipate.

Pain is a hard thing to recall. All my life I've had terrible menstrual periods with bad cramps. I always thought I'd be able to handle labor, because I thought, "I've been able to live through this for twenty years." And if labor was anything like cramps, I'd be able to handle it. Labor is more intense and you don't really know what to expect. Knowing all the things that could happen helps prepare you. Reading books is important, but nothing prepares you fully for the whole experience.

You're going through it alone. I mean you're the one who's having the pain, and you're the one who's going through it, but just having somebody there—I could have done it alone, but I wouldn't have wanted to. Before the birth took place, I wasn't sure my husband would hold up under it, but he did great. And best of all, we created a shared memory, and were able to bond as a couple to our son.

Introduction to Chapter 5

Labor, Delivery, Recovery, and Postpartum Room (LDRP Room)

The LDRP room is an offshoot of the alternative birth center (ABC) room concept, in that instead of moving the mother into the various rooms, the staff comes to the laboring woman, while she stays in one room during all phases of labor, delivery, recovery, and postpartum. This room is a standard-looking labor room, with all the necessary equipment in the one room. There are several differences between them: In the LDRP room, any and all medical intervention is allowed, whereas in the ABC room, intervention is more limited, according to the hospital's protocols. There is more flexibility in the LDRP room, but couples who want as close to a home birth as possible choose the ABC room, which implies less intervention. They are both private rooms, and women stay in either one for their entire stay in the hospital.

Many hospitals have discontinued the use of their ABC room(s), in favor of having all the rooms either LDR (labor, delivery, recovery) or LDRP (labor, delivery, recovery, and postpartum) rooms. Often that means the hospital's obstetric floor has more rooms, but they're smaller, to accommodate more women.

Technical Reference: *Laurence D. Colman, M.D., speacializing in Obstetrics, Gynecology, Infertility, and Endocrinology, Santa Monica, California*

Joan

Joan talks about the birth of her third child, born without any medication in a LDRP room in a local hospital. She compares this birth to her first and second experiences, and shares information about her family situation.

There were a lot of mixed emotions when I decided to have another child. I had two other children from my first marriage. I was raised Catholic, in the midwest, and I was going through guilt and pain because of my divorce and my values. I had to call on all my courage to file for divorce. I never wanted a bad marriage to be the legacy for my kids.

Now I'm happily married to a wonderful man. Things really worked out well for me. My kids adore him. My oldest child is twelve—he's been difficult, but also the most incredible boy I've ever met. And my nine-year-old daughter is "Miss Mellow," a dream child.

The relationship with my second husband has been such a joy! As soon as the divorce was final, I threw out the diaphragm and we were married a month later. I was actually terrified in some ways about whether I could get pregnant this third time, and with a different husband. I come from a very fertile family, but you hear all these things about couples who have difficulties getting pregnant. I never give myself a break. I worried that something dreadful would happen to my body, because in each of my previous pregnancies I gained forty-five pounds and had large babies. I think it's hard on the body, and it's also hard for me to get the weight off.

Anthony was a nine-pound, one-ounce baby, and it was a long labor. My water broke early, and then labor began. I went to the hospital and walked around as much as possible while I was laboring. Then, after three hours of pushing, I couldn't get him out. They almost had to do a C-section, but against everyone's will I pushed him out. I was determined to get him out myself. The recovery was great—after giving birth, I'm higher than a kite!

With my second child, Katie, her birth was a very spiritual experience. I was really in tune with her. I was sure she was going to be a girl and we'd be very close. I had all these fantasies.

When I arrived at the hospital on delivery day, the nurse found out how much weight I gained and was disgusted, putting me down subtly. She was anything but fantastic. In the middle of the hardest part of my labor, she told me my pediatrician just died. She was off the wall, saying hostile and inappropriate things.

I was bound and determined to make it a good experience, so I concentrated on the child within me, and boom! Everything happened quickly and wonderfully after that. Katie was born in the alternative birth center room of a local hospital, at eight o'clock in the morning, and the sun was shining. The sad part was she was born on February 29. I felt like that was a curse, because it would only come around every four years. I thought this would lead to tremendous grief for her and affect her identity.

After Katie's birth, I stayed only one night, because I was concerned about my two-year-old son. When I got home, I realized I should have stayed a little longer in the hospital.

It took me three months to get pregnant the third time, with Steven. The two months before I got pregnant, I felt doom and gloom that I wouldn't be able to get pregnant. Then I was delighted, but also frightened, when I did get pregnant. I was thirty-nine, soon to be forty, and worried about mental retardation. After I had amniocentesis, the fear lifted. But being raised Catholic gave me the notion that God had been so good to me, and there's so much pain and sorrow in the world, why hadn't I suffered any pain and sorrow? I kept thinking—my turn will come. Was I pushing fate to have a third child? I had left my first husband and caused him a lot of pain. To me, it was like I broke one of the Ten Commandments.

My first two births were natural childbirths—I didn't take *any* pain medication. I wanted the same for my third baby. I would never push my luck and have a baby at home. There's too much … that could go wrong. I wouldn't want to jeopardize the health of the child.

I went back to my first obstetrician. The nine months went by quickly—I always feel good when I'm pregnant. The difference with this birth was the labor.

The morning I went into labor, I was getting ready to go to work (I'm a kindergarten teacher). I was making the kids' lunches, and I felt different. With the other two pregnancies, my water broke, and then I went into labor. With this one, I felt cramping. So I called the substitute desk, because I knew I wouldn't be able to teach school that day. I told them I was going into labor or it would start soon.

I took a shower and realized I was in labor. I woke my husband, and told him I was pretty sure I was in labor, but my water hadn't broken yet. I thought we should start timing the contractions. They were coming every minute-and-a-half.

Once they started getting stronger, we called the doctor. I told him this was a strange labor for me ... I was having contractions and my water hadn't broken. I thought I should go to the hospital, but I had to make arrangements for my two big kids to get to school. This was about six-fifteen in the morning, and I was going to take my time getting to the hospital.

As soon as I hung up the phone, my water broke and everything went boom! By six-thirty, my labor was in such full swing, I was out of my mind! I had never gone into labor so quickly. We said good-bye to the kids, and they wished us luck as we walked out to the car. I could barely hang on as we drove to the hospital.

Rodney dropped me off and went to park the car, because he knew I needed to get in as fast as possible. I told them inside, "You better get me in there right away. I'm really in labor." They asked if I needed a wheelchair.

I said, "I hate the thought of going upstairs in a wheelchair, but you better bring one around." They got me in one, in the nick of time, and brought me upstairs.

I was put in a room where I stayed throughout my labor, delivery, recovery, and postpartum [LDRP room]. When they examined me, I was seven centimeters dilated. I was not afraid at that point, but the pain was different and excruciating. I didn't experience a lot of pain with the other two labors. They began more slowly and I was able to cope. My cervix was opening up so fast that it was painful. I kind of lost it—I was sweating, and I didn't know what to do.

I wanted my husband to be involved during the birth, especially since this was his first child. We had gone to a refresher Lamaze class together. He was working long hours, starting his own business, and the refresher was all we had time for.

The nurses were a little surprised too, that it was going so fast, and they went to get the doctor. They called him and told him to come quickly. He's got this calming, feminine quality about him. [He's] very shy at first, but very supportive, assuring me that I can do it. I always feel like I'm seeing my brother when I look at his face.

When my doctor came into the LDRP room, everything went boom! I was ready to push very quickly, and I only had to push for fifteen minutes.

This wonderful nurse helped me when I thought Rodney was a little too rough on me. He said, "Oh come on, you can take this." My body felt like it was out of control.

Rodney said something condescending, and the nurse said very firmly, "Look, you don't know what this is like. You've never been through it." He shut up after that, and looked at me with new eyes.

Steven was in such a hurry to come. Even though there was only fifteen minutes of pushing, Rodney had to help me through it, because the pain was so great. I couldn't move up to bear down. There was another nurse who was very supportive, too.

Steven came out and he was a big baby. He weighed nine pounds, two ounces, and I was on top of the world. I've never had so much energy in my life as after I've pushed my babies out. I was so happy and so relieved to see he was healthy. For me it was a big psychological breakthrough. I felt like—with this birth, I could stop punishing myself.

I did know I was having a boy, and I was glad to have found that out. Rodney said he wanted to find out and I said, "No, I don't want to know." Then he convinced me by saying, "If the doctors are going to know, then we're going to know. We'll be able to plan for it and the two big kids will be more psychologically prepared for that." He certainly had a point. So we did find out the sex of the baby ahead of time.

I felt much closer to this child after he popped out. Through the pregnancy we said, "Hi, Steven," when we talked to him. The gifts I received at the baby showers were bought with a boy in mind. I'm really happy I did that. If it were my first child, I probably wouldn't have done that. Rodney was right—it did get the older kids ready. It was perfect for Anthony to have a baby brother, for a lot of reasons. Basically, everyone we know keeps having girls, and that's always upsetting to him.

For Katie, it would have been threatening to have another girl, so it worked out very well. And I'm just glad I had another child. I'm ready to get pregnant again.

After birth, I had more bleeding than normal, at least according to one of the nurses. That wasn't a major thing. I stayed in the hospital a couple of days. I loved all the tender, loving care all the nurses gave me. I felt like a queen in the hospital.

I was in a larger room for Steven's birth—not as cozy as it was for Anthony's and Katie's births. But they had to have more room here for equipment since it was used for all the phases of labor, delivery, recovery, and postpartum. It's become a trend in hospitals to make all the labor rooms into self-contained LDRP rooms. Women can choose medication, intervention, or they can have a non-medicated birth.

I didn't have that wonderful sunlight streaming in like I had for Katie's birth. There may have been a VCR and a tape player, but we didn't have time to grab music and bring it to the hospital. I didn't even have my bag packed! If it had been a longer labor, I might have thought to bring some music along.

The whole labor was only an hour-and-a-half, from the time I started to feel the cramping until I pushed Steven out. I used the same doctor and the same hospital. He's the kind of doctor you'd want to follow to the ends of the earth—he's that good.

With this birth, the labor and delivery nurses were just fabulous! That first time I felt really bad, because the nurses weren't supportive. I had some friends with me for the first birth, and I didn't want that in this birth. I just wanted my husband with me.

My kids didn't want to be at the birth, and I didn't want them to be there. I mean it's a little grueling to witness birth. It could have been unpleasant or something could have gone wrong. I didn't want to take any chances with that. I wanted to protect them from that experience.

They went to school that morning with notes to the secretaries about the impending birth. Rodney picked them up and brought them to the hospital about three-thirty, to see their new brother. They came into the room and held Steven right away.

Anthony's birth took twenty hours, Katie's was six hours, and Steven's was an hour-and-a-half. I wonder what the next one might be like if I have another child? Rodney and I haven't sat down and talked about it, but in my mind, I'm really ready to get pregnant again.

When I was pregnant at thirty-nine I thought to myself, "I can't go through this again." That was because of the weight gain, since I gained over forty pounds with each pregnancy. It's so hard on my body and it's so difficult to take it off again.

I still had fears this time around, like I was pushing my luck. I had raised these two wonderful children, who were really nice kids, and yet you never know how another one might be. Maybe I'd have a child I wouldn't bond with or wouldn't love. I thought of every possible thing that could go wrong, and then I worried about it.

When Steven was born, I saw birthmarks on his face, and I didn't know where they came from. The only thing I could figure out was when I was in high school I had acne, and I still suffer from the scars. I thought I had passed that on to him. It may seem vain to some people, but I think there's a psychological component to the grief about having acne. I plan on taking my scars off soon with dermabrasion.

I kept seeing his scars and all kinds of stupid, neurotic visions of my son being weird.

The other fear I had was, I had brought these two kids to such a wonderful stage in life, and I had more freedom. Could I go through being tied-down, and that back-breaking work—like getting the baby in and out of the car seat and lugging him around? Also, the crying, and staying up nights, and ear infections. I was really frightened that I would look at this baby and not bond with him. As it turned out, I couldn't have been happier. I wanted to eat him up the minute he popped out! I bonded with him a lot faster than I thought I would. I think it's due to having such a happy marriage and loving myself.

I've always punished myself in life. I've thought of myself as the bad seed—the one who acted out the emotions of the family. I was the rebellious one, who had to carry the load of the family. I beat myself up about that for a long, long time. It got me on a self-destructive path for many years. I was a child of the sixties, and that wasn't an easy time to get through childhood. My father's family was a hard bunch to get through. I felt like, "I wouldn't be able to do this right," as a life script.

I think now, at forty, I'm learning to love myself. During the nine months of pregnancy, I wasn't sure I could give birth as I had with my other two kids. When Steven was born, I thought, "I can do this—I really am a strong woman." Suddenly I was able to validate myself.

[For a long time] I didn't have a higher power in my life, [and] a spiritual life really makes living easier. I've been involved in an alternative lifestyle, by living in a communal house for the past seventeen years. It's been a great lifestyle. One of the best parts is the different role models the children are exposed to. They always have another role model to see ... [and they benefit] by seeing how the other adults respond to them.

The adults in the house take on the responsibilities of parenting all the children, even though we keep within our own families— we respect that. We don't try to rob each other's kids of their allegiance to their parents. We help out with discipline, taking the kids places, baby-sitting, cooking, cleaning.

In a lot of ways, to live in a commune takes more discipline— you can't just leave messes, otherwise you live in a junk pile. We share childcare, cooking, house jobs. We pool money for all the food and the running of the house. We've been together since 1972. We adore the close-knit family we have become, especially since we all live far away from our families of origin. Being part of the commune has been one of the biggest contributors to my growth.

My first two births were Leboyer births. I read Leboyer's book and looked for doctors who would do that kind of birth. When I was interviewing doctors, I met the doctor I chose for all of my births. At that time, I was into doing everything "right and natural." I wanted to do the "in" thing. That was in 1977. The memory of it is very hazy, because that was twelve years ago.

Even though I never had drugs for my births, there's still a part of me that's removed from the scene, to protect the birth. When I had Katie, I watched that birth much more carefully. The doctor gave her a bath after the birth, and that was a good experience.

With this third one, I thought I wasn't going to be masochistic. If I needed to have drugs, because it was a long labor or there was a lot of pain, I would ask for drugs. I was much more realistic about the whole thing. If I needed to have drugs, then "no shame." I had two vaginal births without any drugs, and I didn't need to prove myself in that area.

I didn't ask for a Leboyer bath for my third child, and it wasn't until he popped out that I realized it and wondered if I'd miss it if I didn't have it for Steven. I didn't miss it at all.

I breast-fed all three babies immediately after birth. That's where I have the problem, and that's my shame—I have a lot of trouble nursing. It's so painful for me. My family has very sensitive skin.

The nurses gave me a nipple shield when I had Anthony. I nursed for about three months, and he was not gaining weight as he should, according to the pediatrician who suggested I give it up. I felt badly about that, like I was the biggest failure in the whole world.

Then, with Katie, I was bound and determined to nurse. The pain was so excruciating that I would have drunk a bottle of wine, if I could have, when I nursed her. I called La Leche League and said, "I've got to nurse my baby, I've just got to do it." They sent me this lactation consultant who was really great. She came every day and helped me through it, and I succeeded.

With Steven, I went through the same problem. Every time I nursed, the pain diminished a little bit, but it was much worse than labor. I actually have no pain at all now, because I had the lactation consultant come back and help me position Steven on the breast better, so ... [nursing] didn't hurt.

For me, the LDRP room was very similar to the alternative birth center room (ABC room) I used at the same hospital, many years ago. I liked staying in one room, knowing there were choices of intervention available. The nursing staff was supportive and well-trained—an improvement from the first and second births.

The LDRP rooms look more like hospital rooms than the ABC room did, and that's because there was only one ABC room, and it was furnished differently from the labor rooms. The ABC room had flowered wallpaper, a wooden rocking chair, and a king-size bed. There was no equipment in it, not even a monitor.

There are about twenty LDRP rooms at this hospital, and they look like labor rooms.... They have monitors, and none of the furnishings that were in the ABC room. They have smaller beds, which come apart for delivery—they are a type of birthing bed that modern hospitals are now using.

For women who are presently planning to give birth, the LDRP room is a fine place to have a baby, especially when a woman wants to have a hospital birth, and wants to have the option of intervention and medication.

Introduction to Chapter 6
"Traditional" Labor and Delivery Rooms

This "traditional" type of birth has been used by mothers since the turn of the century. The mother in our story decided to use epidural anesthesia as medication for her traditional birth. It allowed her to be alert and participate in the delivery, yet minimize the side-effects frequently suffered from either spinal anesthesia or general anesthesia.

When a woman is admitted to the hospital in labor, there are standard procedures for her to follow. Most hospitals require the laboring woman to be escorted to the maternity section in a wheelchair. It's not because she isn't able to walk; it's for insurance purposes.

*In the labor room, the first thing she does after she changes her clothes and puts on a hospital gown is empty her bowels and bladder, and provide a urine specimen. She has her blood pressure checked, [gets] an internal exam to determine cervical effacement or dilation; and then, if in fact she is in actual labor, she's hooked up to an **external fetal heart monitor**. This machine will monitor her baby's heart rate, and show the frequency and size of her uterine contractions. Two belts each with a metal disc attached, are placed around the woman's abdomen, to pick up the baby's heart rate and the uterine contractions, and show their electrical impulses on the monitor's screen. The general rule is for the hospital to do a "strip reading" for twenty to thirty minutes. A labor nurse will watch the changes taking place on the monitor for that time, and evaluate the woman's progress.*

The woman will continue laboring in the labor room until she reaches full dilation of her cervix, or ten centimeters. When she is fully dilated, and ready to push, she is transferred onto a gurney and taken to the delivery room. This means she has to move onto another bed (the gurney, in this case) while she's in very active labor.

Once in the delivery room, the doctor and nurses assist the woman to push her baby out. She is generally in a sitting position, because this position is more efficient for bringing the baby out and the baby receives more oxygen when the mother is upright. A common position for delivery is sitting, with a nurse on either side of the woman holding up one of her legs.

After the baby is delivered and brought into the nursery, the mother expels the placenta, and then she is transferred to a recovery room. In the course of her birth, she has been in at least three rooms, and will go into a fourth, a private or shared room, for her postpartum stay.

Technical Reference: *Laurence D. Colman, M.D., specializing in Obstetrics, Gynecology, Infertility, and Endocrinology, Santa Monica, California*

Tracy

Tracy is forty-six-years-old, with two grown daughters. In her second marriage, she becomes pregnant for the second time, and the amniocentesis shows a healthy fetus.

When I found out I was pregnant, I was pretty concerned about it. I think the trauma of having a baby is stressful on the body, and maybe the older you get, the more stressful it is. I wanted the most painless birth I could have. I even considered having a cesarean, except that I found out the recuperation period is longer, and it's no less stressful on the body. So for me, having a cesarean would not have traumatized me.

The reason I wanted to have a pain-free birth was based on the fact that I had had two extremely painful births and I didn't think it was anything to be proud of. I think painless is better. I mean, the object is to have a healthy baby, and if I could do it painlessly— wonderful!

My husband [never]did . . . want me to have natural childbirth. . . . He thought it would be bad for the baby. We were taking Lamaze classes and they were stressing no medication. However, being older and wiser, I felt like I just wouldn't let anyone deter me from that [medication].

I told my husband the classes would serve as a support group, . . .[and we could] learn the breathing, [to use] until the time came when I could have a regional anesthetic. The information was really interesting. It was nice, but I never for a minute intended to have the baby naturally.

It was almost a struggle this time to convince everyone that I wanted an epidural and there was no way I was going to even try not having it. The doctor said, "Well let's see if you need it."

59

And I said, "I don't care if I do or don't. I want it." I was adamant about having an epidural as soon as I reached five centimeters dilation. By the time I was in labor, everyone knew that's the way it was going to be. And the nursing staff was absolutely wonderful and supportive.

If epidural anesthesia is used, the lower half of the body is numbed, however the woman is able to move those affected areas. The woman is prepped before the epidural, her back swabbed with an antiseptic solution, and then draped with sheets. Epidural anesthesia spreads through the epidural space, to the nerves, surrounding the spinal column. As the levels of anesthesia increase, the nerves are blocked from sending pain impulses to the brain. An epidural takes from ten to twenty minutes to become effective, and can be increased in length as needed.

There are drawbacks to using this type of anesthesia. It is difficult to predict how effective an epidural will be for an individual. Sometimes numbing is spotty, meaning there is partial feeling in the incision site. Then an additional type of anesthesia is given. Incorrect placement of an epidural injection can cause "partial or total spinal anesthesia," although that rarely happens. In a partial spinal, the woman will have a "spinal headache" unless she stays lying down for at least twenty-four hours. If she has "total spinal anesthesia," the woman's breathing can be unsteady, so she is usually given a general anesthetic, as well. Then the anesthesiologist can regulate her breathing.

Recovery after epidural anesthesia is normally tolerated well, with some pain medication. There may be three separated sources of pain: the site of the incision; the uterus contracting; and possibly pain under the shoulder blade, caused by air trapped under the diaphragm during delivery.
—**Laurence Colman, M.D.,** Santa Monica, California

My experience with my first birth was so different. It was almost twenty-five years ago. I don't remember having a choice, or anything, [about] whether I wanted medication or not. I had not taken classes; I knew nothing.

My first husband was a doctor, and he kept telling me about the women in China who went into the fields to have their babies. Then they went right back to work. I went in not expecting birth to be a big deal, because I was going to be like Chinese peasant women who have their babies in fields.

I wasn't prepared for a lot of pain. What I remember was the long labor which was horrendously painful. I asked for medication and was given Percodan to "cut the contractions."

I didn't feel it "cutting" at all. I'd have given anything for medication. I also remember being left alone in the labor room. It was really a terribly lonely, painful, awful experience. I didn't complain, because I thought that's the way it's supposed to be, except I begged for more medication and did not get it. Then, when the baby was being born, they gave me something and I fell asleep at that moment. I missed the thrill of seeing my baby being born!

After I woke up, I didn't dwell on the fact that the birth had been unpleasant. It's only in retrospect, twenty-five years later, when I see what the difference is, that I can look back and say, "That shouldn't have happened." Maybe I'm a little bitter about that experience.

When I had my second baby, four years later, it was better. The staff was friendlier, but I was still alone in the Labor Room. I was given some medication because I don't seem to remember much of the birth. It wasn't particularly bad or good. I remember some nice people.

This recent pregnancy was very different from my others. I had chorionic villus sampling (CVS) testing to verify, early on, that this baby is healthy.

During this test, a fine, hollow tube (cannula) is introduced into the uterus through the vagina and cervix, guided by an ultrasound scan, and some chorionic villus tissue is suctioned out. This tissue sticks out from the maternal side of the developing placenta, and samples of it can be analyzed for genetic and metabolic defects, including Down's syndrome, sickle-cell anemia, and Tay-Sachs disease. The advantage of this test over amniocentesis is that it can be done between the sixth and tenth week, and the results are available in twenty-four hours—rather than amnio at sixteen weeks and waiting two to three weeks for results.
    —**Laurence D. Colman, M.D.,** Santa Monica, California

I later chose the doctor who gave me the test as my obstetrician, because he seemed very warm and competent. I liked him through the entire pregnancy. Going in, the only thing I was afraid of was I wouldn't get the epidural when I wanted it, but that didn't happen. It worked out fine.

In our Lamaze course, there was such a bias against medication. I think that's a crime toward women. The teacher implied that you shouldn't feel like a failure if you have to use medication. But by saying that, it was implied that the best way was without medication. I don't see how you could possibly say, assuming it's not going to harm the baby—which an epidural definitely does not, that it's better one way or another.

I think women have enough things to prove. The object of a birth is to have a healthy baby and a healthy mother, not to see that you can get through it without drugs.

If you want to prove yourself, climb a mountain, get a Ph.D.—there's a million things you can do. Don't wreck your birth experience because you did or didn't use drugs.

As it turned out, the experience was pure joy! I knew when I went into the hospital that I was going to have epidural anesthesia at the earliest possible moment.

The nurse was completely supportive and worked with me in my decision. The doctor was there, and my husband was there for the whole birth. I had the epidural, and it was great! I felt I was participating more in the birth because I wasn't wrapped up in the pain.

I was able to see my baby being born, as he came out. I was able to push, although I didn't know when to push. Everyone in the room was saying, "Okay, one, two, three, push!" It was like a cheering squad.

For this third baby, it was a good twelve hours of labor. It was about twenty-four hours for my first. This was still long. I would not have wanted to go through it without medication.

I remember feeling much better after the birth. With the first one, I thought I could just pop out of bed, but I felt too weak to get up without falling down.

With this one, when I was back in my room and I had to get up, I got up cautiously and I was fine. I walked right into the bathroom.

I think going through a lot of stress and pain definitely has a depleting effect on your body. It has to, because of all the hormones and chemicals that are released through pain.

I would definitely encourage a woman in her forties, as I was this third time, to go ahead and have a baby. Even though I was afraid of birth defects, having given up a fetus with Down's syndrome that was discovered through amniocentesis, it was not enough to stop me from having a baby.

I was concerned about any general birth defects the baby might have. When my doctor said the chances were no higher for birth defects when the woman was in her forties than a woman in her twenties, with the exception of Down's syndrome, I didn't believe it. I still worried, even after I had the CVS test, when I knew the baby did not have Down's syndrome.

For my first and second babies, I was twenty-two and twenty-six, and now I don't think there was that much difference, physically. I had a little more problem with loose ligaments this time, during the last trimester. That's all though. I worked until the last day. It wasn't a traumatic pregnancy at all.

I think there's absolutely nothing compared to having a baby. I would have missed so much if I hadn't had a child. I can't imagine a woman who doesn't want a baby. Even if they don't want a baby, they'll want it after it's born. Women who choose not to have children are just missing the world.

With the advances in technology, there's no reason to lead women into believing they're better off without medication. I think it's a shame that women have been taught to avoid pain medication. It's a trick—I just don't know what to say about it.

And the same with cesareans. Maybe they're doing too many of them, I don't know. But cesareans are saving an awful lot of babies' lives, and probably a lot of women's lives, too. I wish women wouldn't be so suspicious of modern medicine.

I know there are a lot of women who could give me the opposite view of modern medicine, but I'm thankful at age forty-six for the CVS test, which can be performed between the sixth and tenth week, and after sixteen weeks the blood test for spina bifida.

Spina bifida is a neural tube defect in the baby, where part of the spinal column protrudes from the back.
—**Your Baby, Your Way,** by Sheila Kitzinger, Pantheon 1987

Find out who the head labor nurse is, and talk to her about what you want. That's probably more important than just hearing from the doctor, "Yes, we can do that for you." You'll find out that the head nurse has a lot of control, especially if the doctor is not available at the time.

It's important for women to know what goes on in the labor room. Knowing what your rights are is critical, so you can express yourself, and if you're not able to your husband can speak for you.

I think it's very important to feel that your husband is going to support you in whatever you want. But don't go in thinking the whole staff is against you. They're not, they're really for you. It really disturbs me to hear how awful all these people are. I don't think they're awful; they're doing their jobs.

Women need to go over their birth plan with their doctors or midwives before the birth, to find out that it's a workable plan. Sometimes, women think the doctors are breaking their promise when, in fact, they might be on a different track from the woman. Many go in with a chip on their shoulder. They think, "Modern medicine is terrible and sterile, and the staff is terrible," so they find what they're looking for. It's a self-fulfilling prophecy.

With regard to pain during labor, I actually was walking our dogs and my water broke. Just before it broke, I had a lot of pressure down there. I thought I was feeling pressure, but it was really hurting, and I still thought it was pressure. It wasn't anything unbearable; I wasn't panicked.

One of the reasons I wasn't too worried about the pain was I felt pretty confident that they'd give me something to stop ... [it]. If I had to go through it another few hours, it wasn't terrible. It didn't seem like it would be interminable. However, I was in a hurry to get it over with. I had been going around with small contractions for a week.

It worked out quite well because the baby was born on a Friday. As a dentist, I don't work Fridays, so I worked through Thursday, and I was able to finish up all the root canals and everything else, and sort of leave with a clear slate—not having things hanging over.

It did take me longer to take off the weight I put on during the pregnancy, and to get back in shape, than with my other two pregnancies. With those, the weight sort of fell off really fast. With this one, it went down pretty quickly, but then there was a residual five to ten pounds that took quite a long time to come off.

There was another decision I made, which I had a hard time about. I hadn't nursed my other children, and I didn't want to nurse this one. I don't like nursing, and I know some people might think I'm a bad mother because I chose not to do that. Meanwhile, I have two adult kids who are very nice [and] normal. I don't think they were deprived.

I feel the same non-conformity when it comes to pain. Women say that even the day after they have their babies, they're ready to do it again. It's like amnesia about their pain, but I did remember how painful it was. I never dwelled on it afterwards. Once I had the baby I was happy, and the pain happened a long time ago. But when I was faced with having another child, the pain memory came back. Since I had a choice for the third birth, I chose medication to overcome the pain.

Introduction to Chapter 7

Vacuum Extraction Delivery

The vacuum extractor is an electronically operated machine. Attached to the machine is a hose, at the end of which is a metal or plastic cup about four inches in diameter which is placed on the baby's head. When the machine is turned on, suction runs through the tube and into the cup, drawing part of the baby's head within it. Since the head is the largest part of the infant, when it is pulled through the opening, the body easily follows.

Many obstetricians prefer vacuum extraction in circumstances where forceps could be used. As with forceps, the head is rotated into a better position for delivery by using the extractor.

The advantages of this method over using forceps are that it is an easier method of extraction than forceps, and there is little risk of damaging the baby. By this method, a characteristic, puffy, rounded area on the baby's head is produced, rather than marks left from forceps, which are noticeable at first, but disappear within a day or two.

*The disadvantages of **vacuum extraction** are that a vacuum extraction procedure takes a few minutes longer than a forceps procedure, and there is possible risk of blood blisters or tentorial tears.*

Many doctors today prefer the vacuum extractor over forceps—it takes less skill. Also, newer doctors going through medical school today are not given much practical training in using forceps—it's becoming a lost art in obstetrics. Unless a doctor has been well-trained in the use of forceps, he'll probably avoid using them, and use the extractor instead. If that is unsuccessful, he'll perform a cesarean section as a last resort.

Technical Reference: *Laurence D. Colman, M.D., specializing in Obstetrics, Gynecology, Infertility and Endocrinology, Santa Monica, California*

Sheila

Sheila decided to use regular labor and delivery rooms to give birth to her first child because more options would be available to her. She expected problems, and worried that she'd panic when she started labor. It turned out better than she anticipated.

I had just turned thirty-four when my baby was born. I had no intention of being a martyr, but I wanted the birth to be as drug-free as possible. I was willing to have an epidural or whatever was recommended, and thought I'd probably end up wanting some kind of pain-killer.

In our Bradley course, the teacher thoroughly explained the kinds of drugs and interventions we could use, and what the risks were. She wasn't promoting drug-free births, but rather helping us become well-informed. If the doctor suggested a particular drug or intervention, she wanted us to know what was involved. I read a lot, too, but the Bradley class was very helpful for both my husband and me.

I don't think you're ever truly prepared for childbirth. Each experience is new and different. Nobody can tell you what it's like. Since this was my first child, I really had no idea what to expect. From all I had read, from the films I saw, and from the birthing course, I expected it to be a difficult process. I wondered if I would say, "I can't stand it. Give me whatever is necessary to get rid of this pain." I wanted to be like the women in the films who managed so well, but I was afraid I wouldn't be.

We decided to have the baby in a hospital. Rather than use the the hospital's alternative birth center room, we decided to use a regular labor room since this gave us the option of having drugs if I felt I needed them.

Before I went into labor, I worried that things wouldn't go right. I didn't have anything specific in my mind—I'm just such a worrier. I had that common fear of a lot of women that I might not make it to the hospital in time. I worried about what the labor would be like and how long it would last.

I went to the hospital with "false labor" because I was having contractions every thirty minutes for several hours. The contractions lasted forty-five seconds to a minute—longer than "real labor" contractions, which in the earliest stage last ten to fifteen seconds. They gave me morphine because I wasn't dilating, and sent me home to get some sleep. I called a friend and told her, "This is the worst experience of my life!" The nausea and vomiting from the morphine was really bothering me. When I talked to her the day after the baby was born, I said, "That wasn't so bad!"

I was having what I thought were gas pains—like indigestion—that hit about every twenty minutes, when we went to the hospital at about midnight on Monday, but by three or four in the morning I hadn't progressed at all.

The doctor said, "You need sleep and the baby needs sleep." He said the morphine will either stop the false labor or it will make things progress. It stopped the contractions and allowed me to sleep.

Wednesday morning my water broke and we returned to the hospital. I had slept most of the night, but I was aware of some contractions while I slept. I wasn't in pain so I slept through them. After my water broke, my husband wanted to time the contractions. I wanted to go to the hospital, and became rather irritated. I was having a hard time getting through the contractions unless I had total concentration. When we got to the hospital I was eight centimeters dilated.

My husband said I was temperamental. I kept telling him we should go to the hospital, and he wanted to continue timing the contractions. Since we had already been sent home once, he wanted to make sure we were far enough along with labor before returning to the hospital. I've talked to other women who also became obnoxious during labor even though they are usually even-tempered and mild-mannered.

An hour after we were in the hospital, I felt like I wanted to push. I was examined and told I could begin. I pushed and pushed and pushed. That was the hard part. They told me I'd find pushing a relief—I found it really painful. I tried every position I could get into.

After two hours, I was exhausted. The doctor decided I wouldn't be able to deliver the baby without some help. So they moved me to the delivery room to try the vacuum extractor. If that didn't work he would try forceps, and if that didn't work I would have to have a cesarean, which I didn't want. They tried the vacuum extractor and it was painful. I was given spinal anesthesia to help relax the muscles and then I didn't feel any pain.

My husband was really good about helping me push, and became quite a pro at timing my contractions. The hardest part of the birth was pushing. I knew when I had to push 'cause I could feel when the baby was beginning to move in a wave motion. Then when I stopped pushing, I felt pain. After all the energy it took to keep pushing, I was exhausted. Since so many women enjoy this part of childbirth, their babies must have been in a better position for them to push than mine was. He was a big baby and I'm not very big. The doctor finally got the baby's head in the proper position. It had been tilted back, and this slowed down his journey through the birth canal and caused me a lot of pain. Maybe I was just too tired to help him come through.

The spinal didn't hurt at all and, after two tries with the extractor, he was born. I wanted them to adjust the mirror so I could watch the delivery, but the anesthesiologist said I wouldn't be able to see the mirror anyway. I was sorry I couldn't see him being delivered. I heard everyone yelling and screaming. My husband saw him immediately. He was placed on my stomach right away, but I wish I could have seen him come into the world. That would have made birth even more wonderful. I also missed the sensation of actually feeling him being born. He weighed nine pounds, three ounces, and was twenty-two inches long.

I completely trusted everyone there. I was in control and believed everything would work out fine, which it did, but it was not what I anticipated. I didn't know myself as well as I thought I did. Giving birth was a mind-expanding experience which had a profound effect on me, and it made me feel more capable as a woman.

I expected to panic, but I didn't. I managed. It wasn't as bad as I thought. The pain was tolerable. I loved my doctor, and I felt like I was getting excellent care. I trusted him—everything he said, and all the decisions were made together. The nurses were great and my husband was just terrific.

Maybe if I had exercised during my pregnancy, like I was supposed to, I would have had enough stamina to push him out. I've thought a lot about this as I'm sure many women do when their childbirth experience is not what they expected.

I could have ended up with a cesarean if I'd had a doctor who was less patient or less skilled. My doctor did everything possible to avoid an unnecessary C-section. I'm grateful he took the time to try the vacuum extractor before using forceps or performing a cesarean.

I was lucky to have had the birthing experience I did. I felt in complete control while I was in labor—I felt fine.

What stood out about my birth experience was how incredible it was to have such a big, healthy, beautiful baby. It was a miracle! Suddenly there he was and I could hardly believe it! It was hard to comprehend that he had really come from me!

The more educated you are about childbirth, the better. I got all the information I could from friends and professionals, and from books they recommended. We determined which car seat was best to buy long before the baby arrived [essential because you can't take the baby home from the hospital without one] and we attended Baby Care class. [Baby Care is a Red Cross course that gives instruction for couples about bathing, feeding, and postpartum care for the baby and mother.]

I think you have to be a well-informed consumer in all medical issues, and especially where childbirth is concerned. It's important to be aware of what the ramifications are regarding the decisions you and your doctor make, and feel comfortable with your doctor and with the decisions made. It's not that you have to go along with them. At first I didn't want to have the morphine, but after I had the medication, I thought it was a good decision.

I had no idea what it was going to be like to be a mother until I actually had to do it. Even though my brother has three kids, and I spend a lot of time with them, it's not the same. I've had as much preparation as anybody, probably more. I've been around kids a lot. I have a degree in child development and I've worked at pre-school so I know what a baby does. But when it was my own baby, and I brought him home, I didn't know what I was doing.

Fortunately, the last Baby Care class dealt with what you do once you bring the baby home, and that was very helpful. I had imagined a cooing, gurgling little bundle of joy, but she set the scene with a colicky, fussy baby, crying all night—not all fun and games. As it turned out, the first six weeks were dreadful—our baby cried all the time!

It would have been nice to have family living nearby. I especially miss them at a special time like this. They'd be better able to share our joy if they could see and hold the baby.

One thing that has helped has been attending a support group with mothers and newborns. The group provides contact with other mothers and babies, and we get a chance to discuss the problems and rewards of being new mothers. We hear common concerns, and realize we're not alone. The emotional support from this group of mothers really helps.

I take the responsibility of motherhood seriously, as I think all mothers should, and I don't have any regrets about having this baby. But before jumping into such a life-long committment, it's important to be absolutely sure you want a baby. Your life is never the same again, and the responsibility can be overwhelming—even though you wanted a baby more than anything in the world.

Part II

CESAREAN BIRTH

Cesarean Births Ten Years Apart

In the following story, a woman has two very different experiences with her first and second cesarean births. The births took place in 1976 and in 1986—the ten years between accounted for the change in practices that occurred.

In the mid to end of the seventies, hospitals were beginning to allow husbands into operating rooms, when a C-section was being performed. They began offering cesarean preparation classes, for couples who were having a scheduled cesarean section, and they were also being suggested for couples who wanted to prepare for that possibility.

In 1976, the mother received a knock-out dose of anesthetic, through a mask over her face. She was completely out while the doctor closed the incisions (one in the uterus and one in the abdomen), and she was pretty much out of it for the next twelve to twenty-four hours. For a "scheduled cesarean," a sleeping pill was given the night before surgery, making her less conscious of the birth process the next morning. She remained in the hospital longer, and couldn't get up to walk as soon as she could in 1986.

Even for an "emergency cesarean," an epidural block is usually the only anesthetic given, so the mother is conscious for the entire birth. Attending medical professionals seem more relaxed and assured, than in '76, less fearful of malpractice suits. Husbands may stay with their wives, and are offered the privilege of cutting the umbilical cord, giving their newborns their first freedom. Often, siblings can hold and bond with the baby immediately, in the recovery room, with Mom and Dad there, too. The new mother stays in the hospital about four days, and is walking around the day after giving birth.

Most cesareans are unexpected, so it's valuable for couples to learn at least a little about what to expect if surgery is required. The typical class is three hours long, and if held in a hospital, a maternity tour is often included. The couple can see the operating, recovery, and postpartum rooms, as well as the nursery. Many hospitals require the father or coach to attend the Cesarean Preparation Class, in order to be allowed into the operating room, as a support to you, and as a way to feel connected to the birth of his baby.

Unless a cesarean section is an emergency, due to hemorrhage, prolapsed cord, or fetal distress, there will be time for a member of your medical team to explain the reason surgery is necessary.

Technical Reference: *The Birth Center, Salee Berman, C.N.M., and Victor Berman, M.D., Prentice Hall Press, 1986*

Mary

Mary has two daughters, ten years apart. She describes the differences between the two births, and the challenges she faced with infertility.

My first daughter was born when I was thirty-two. She weighed nine pounds, ten ounces, and it was a week-delayed birth. My wonderful gynecologist had seen a lot of women suffer through long labors, only to finally require a cesarean delivery. Those ladies were physical wrecks, and I imagine they paid the price for a long time. I was thrilled with my doctor for saying, "I'm not going to put you through that." A month before my due date, he told me my baby probably couldn't be born vaginally. As it turned out, I had some contractions, but I never dilated.

He did a C-section at nine o'clock on a Saturday morning, which was quite convenient. My best friend's daughter was born on March 8, and when the doctor asked me when I'd like to have the C-section, I told him on Saturday, March 8, not expecting him to do it on a Saturday, but he said that was fine.

Interestingly enough, I never felt any regret about it—no one talked about the disappointment of having a cesarean birth. My mother, who's a nurse, was hoping it would be a C-section, because I was huge and she was very concerned. She had a difficult forceps birth with her first child, my brother. Mom had geared me to think about a C-section, but not in any negative way. When the doctor said that's what they were going to do, I wasn't terribly concerned. So many of my friends, in their thirties, were having C-sections.

The experience itself wasn't pleasant. I took all the Lamaze classes, and practiced all the exercises and the breathing. But I wasn't disappointed at not being able to put it to use. The C-section saved me a lot of work.

My roommate in the hospital was with me only the night before surgery, but she was so helpful that I'll never forget her, and always be grateful for her description of each step that would take place in my cesarean. She was a nurse at another hospital, and had just had her third C-section. I was sorry to see her go home the next morning and leave me alone.

Of course, another thing I didn't like was that they didn't allow husbands in the operating room. They gave me spinal anesthesia, and later I had a headache from it. As soon as the baby was born, they put me out to stitch up my uterus. I woke up in the recovery room, without any of the fun or excitement that took place in the second birth. I was relieved to know our first baby was healthy, but I missed seeing her right after the delivery. In fact, I didn't see her until noon the next day—twenty-seven hours later. It was really not bonding like the classic thing. I think there's a lot to be said about letting that baby come into the family, and letting everybody hold it—especially the dad.

In the sixth or seventh month of my second pregnancy—with my second child—my hairdresser asked if I was excited about the birth. I told her the only part I didn't like was being put under. She said, "They don't do that anymore."

I went right home and called my doctor to confirm that. I had no idea that had changed in the ten years.

For the second birth, the doctor thought it safest for me to have a C-section, especially because I had lost two babies since my first child was born. The surgery was scheduled for July 21.

I went into labor a week before that, and arrived at the hospital in the middle of the night. The doctor performed an unscheduled cesarean and she was born between three and four in the morning.

It was a much easier birth—a piece of cake. My husband was in the operating room, and he cut the cord. It was such a difference …as soon as I was moved from the operating room to the recovery room, my ten-year-old daughter held her new sister.

I had no qualms about the baby being born by cesarean. I did go into a more defined labor, although I never dilated. In the second pregnancy, even though I was ten years older, I felt more physically fit than during my first pregnancy. I taught an aerobics class during this second pregnancy, and I had a much quicker recovery after the second surgery. I'm a great believer in getting right up and walking, as soon as possible after surgery.

I had a young roommate the second time, who could have been my daughter—she was twenty. She had a normal birth, but wouldn't take any drugs because she was terrified of becoming addicted. It was a big mistake, because she was in too much pain to get out of bed, and she had a vaginal delivery.

What I tell women who are having abdominal surgery is, "Take the drugs or medications they give you while you're in the hospital, and get up and walk and walk and walk. You can't walk if you don't take the pain medicine and you are in pain. Don't be a martyr."

There's a phenomenon men will never comprehend, and that's knowing there's a baby who has to come out. Before I ever gave birth, I had this apprehension about not understanding how that was going to be. With the second baby, I just knew it would happen, and I didn't think about it as much. I don't like hospitals and surgery, but I was resolved about it, because in the end I'd have my baby. It made a difference that I was holding my husband's hand and looking into his eyes during the surgery the second time. It was more of a bond than just an antiseptic experience.

I actually wasn't aware of what they were doing when they were getting me ready for the anesthesia. They ask you to roll into a ball as much as you can, so the anesthesiologist can insert the needle in the correct place in the spine for an epidural. I really like when doctors explain what they're doing beforehand. I'd always rather hear it than not, because then I can deal with it.

My husband wasn't allowed in the operating room until after the anesthesia had been administered. I know some doctors who will allow the husbands in as soon as the woman is wheeled into the operating room. Had that been the case, my husband would have held my hand and I would have been less scared. I did ask the anesthesiologist, "Will someone hold my hand?"

He said, "We're too busy to hold your hand."

My second birth would have been enhanced if my husband could have been with me when they were giving me the anesthesia. It would have helped calm me down. It worked against the anesthesiologist not to have him there.

I felt fabulous, both physically and mentally, after the second birth. The first one was depressing, because I couldn't see my baby for twenty-seven hours. Neither baby was a good nurser. I believe they gave my first one sugar water, because it took her awhile to adjust to sucking on the breast.

The first and second births were very different experiences. Ironically, I was in better physical shape at forty-two, than at thirty-two. I was not an exercise person in my thirties. For both my pregnancies, I gained a ton of weight, which seems to be my pattern.

The age of the mother isn't as important as her health and physical condition. I wouldn't have any qualms if I were to have a baby now at forty-four, as long as I had amniocentesis so I wouldn't have to worry for nine months if the baby was healthy or not.

I chose to have a roommate ... the second ... [time], because in my first birth I stayed in a single room after ... [delivering]. I felt lonely and I thought it'd be fun to share thoughts and feelings with another new mother. I got the wrong roommate though, and it was a terrible experience.

For two hours, I had a roommate who would have been great. She was getting ready to go home, but I think our babies would have been friends forever. When my mother had my brother, she met another woman in the hospital, and they're still good friends to this day.

I think it was a mistake, again on the hospital's part, to put a twenty-year-old vaginal delivery, with a forty-two-year-old C-section. Masses of people came in and out of the room to see her, and she had her baby brought to her when I was trying to sleep that first night. I spent most of the time in the breast-feeding room, since the situation was so intolerable.

I think that's something women need to decide—whether to have a private room or share a room. I was really naive.... I didn't realize, until much later, how women look at rooms in the hospital before they have their babies. They know which room to request in advance.

On the second birth, I was so fortunate. I called at eleven-thirty at night, on my doctor's exchange, and he was at the hospital with another woman in labor. My baby was delivered while this woman was still laboring. Unfortunately, she had to have a C-section many hours later. She wanted to avoid a C-section, and tried as long as possible. I guess one never knows if it's possible to make it through a long labor, unless one tries.

I did appreciate not having to go through labor, especially in the first birth, because … [the baby] was very, very big. I think I was very lucky. I had two different doctors. The magic of an obstetrician is they read what you need. They were there for me, and I didn't ask them a lot of questions.

I read many books about the Lamaze method, for my first birth.

For the second baby, I didn't read as much about birth. We did use the book, *A Child Is Born,* by Lennart Nilson. In fact, we had two copies of it, one for ourselves and one for our daughter. We loved to look at all the prenatal photographs during my pregnancy.

I don't know how you can feel fulfilled as a woman if you haven't had a child. I think it's the most productive, wonderful thing to be able to nurture a growing person. I have known friends who have changed their whole way of life while carrying their babies. When I've been pregnant, I've been at my healthiest— getting more sleep, eating a better diet. I wish more mothers did that. I would have missed a lot if I hadn't had any children.

I went through seven years of fertility work to get the first baby, which cost me my first marriage. I was always at the clinics. I had a laparoscopy, [had] taken Clomid and Pergonal—I really paid my dues. To this day, they're not sure what triggered the pregnancy of my first daughter, since I took Pergonal in February and became pregnant in June. The drugs are only supposed to affect the current month and possibly the following month.

The same thing with the second baby—I was remarried, and we tried and tried, and then I had a tubal pregnancy. The doctor did some exploratory work when the embryo had to be removed from my fallopian tubes. I became pregnant again, and that ended in a miscarriage. I was able to get pregnant a third time, and that resulted in Emily.

Becoming pregnant was the most important thing in my life, in my late twenties. I was used to getting whatever I wanted from hard work or diligence, but I could not get a baby. I think, had I not been able to have a baby, I would have altered my lifestyle. I was always around kids, and had a lot of love from children, but it wasn't the same as having my own.

The birth experience seems to be when you hear the baby cry. I remember it indelibly with both children. I suppose it's also when the doctor says, "It's a girl, and she's fine." With my first daughter, Allison, they said, "It's a girl and she's beautiful," and then they put me under.

I think it's an interesting question for a C-section mother— When does the birth experience begin? To me, it was the crying of the baby and the emotions of the doctor. I don't relate at all to women who feel they've missed something because they didn't have a vaginal birth. From my point of view, I'd rather have the baby than the experience anytime.

I think there's a kind of "Purple Badge of Courage" for women who have had a C-section—it's major surgery, and [through] every minute of the recovery, I thought it was ... worth it. I've had other surgeries in my life, but after those procedures I didn't have a product as a result.

The best way to prepare a woman who is going to have a C-section would be to take her through the process, step-by-step. I'd encourage her to take the sleeping pill the night before, so she is well-rested. She should take pain medication, so she can get up and walk once she's had the surgery. She'll feel better when she walks, and then she'll recover more quickly. Then she can be a good mother.

When a woman is having something other than a normal vaginal birth, she might want to consider having a private room. One of the nurses asked me ... [if I wanted a private room] when she knew I was scheduled to have a cesarean, and I should have picked up on ... [it].

My second marriage was so wonderful! I think that enhanced the whole experience of the second birth. I think birth is very much a mother and child experience, although I was delighted to share it with my husband. Perhaps through Lamaze classes and a vaginal birth there can be more of a shared experience. The stories I hear, though, are not quite like that. Husbands sometimes faint, or aren't the best at coaching. Yet I'm glad the father is included more at births. They can't understand the kicking and the movement that mothers feel all those months. It's a private dance one does with her baby. The mother expects the father to love that baby instantly, but he's not had the nine months of bonding in the way that she has.

After my first was born, and I came home from the hospital, I missed the kicking that went on during the pregnancy. We were bonded through that, and I didn't feel the same connection when I first brought her home.

With the second baby, I had to resurrect my Lamaze. We went to the market at six o'clock in the evening while I was in labor. By the time we got to the hospital, I could see the rise and fall of the contractions on the monitor, and there were *high* peaks. I had to do Lamaze breathing through them, so I used the information from the classes.

I felt so fortunate, because with me it was a total miracle that I could have another child. I knew my second husband, Jim, wanted a baby, but he knew there was a chance we wouldn't be able to have one.

We were married in the summer of eighty-two. Around August I went to a fertility specialist. He was cute with me and said, "At thirty, it's okay, at thirty-five it's harder, and at forty there's such a slight chance of things working in your favor." My track record wasn't too good after having my first baby. I accepted the fact we might not have any more babies.

When I had the tubal pregnancy, I got so excited—I thought it was a pregnancy that would be successful. I wound up in the hospital. That was in the fall of eighty-two. In the spring of eighty-three, I was pregnant again, and I eventually miscarried. That was such a heartbreak! Then in the fall of eighty-three, I was pregnant again and I was just ecstatic, but also scared to death because of the prior experiences.

When you're young, you just don't think of not being able to get pregnant. You want a baby and you think it will just happen. I would say that probably one of the most heartbreaking kinds of people are infertile couples. I'm so happy to have my two precious girls!

Introduction to Chapter 9

Emergency Cesarean Birth

(Please also read "Introduction to Chapters 11 and 12.")

Before a woman undergoes an emergency cesarean, she is given oxygen through a mask, to increase the oxygen circulating in her blood, which in turn gives more oxygen to the baby. By relaxing, and breathing as normally as possible with the mask on, the oxygen is given very quickly.

Then, an injection of sodium pentothal (the most common narcotic used for general anesthesia) is added to the woman's IV, and she is completely asleep in fifteen to twenty seconds. She's not actually unconscious, but she is asleep, making it easier for the anesthetic to be administered. A second injection in the IV contains a muscle relaxant. The entire body becomes relaxed, and reduces the amount of anesthetic and narcotics needed for surgery.

Since the woman is temporarily paralyzed, a rubber tube is inserted into her throat to help regulate breathing. A mixture of oxygen and nitrous oxide is given, either through the tube or through a mask. The gases are inhaled into the lungs and absorbed into the blood. As the blood circulates through the body to the brain, in sufficient amounts, it causes total unconsciousness.

*General anesthesia has more risks than local anesthesia. One of the serious risks to the mother is that she might vomit and ingest liquid into the lungs. Even if she hasn't eaten for many hours, it is possible for some food to be left in the stomach. Eliminating much of this risk is a tube called an **endotracheal tube**, passing through the larynx and into the trachea, which leads directly to the lungs. Anesthesiologists now place this tube as a standard procedure with general anesthesia, to block entrance to the lungs and suction off fluid if the woman vomits during surgery.*

The incision in the uterus is closed with dissolvable stitches, and the incision in the abdomen is generally closed with staples, which are removed in a couple days. The placenta is taken out, along with the baby.

After surgery, when the woman wakes up from general anesthesia, it's likely she will feel a certain amount of confusion. She may come in and out of consciousness, and find it difficult to reconstruct the sequence of events that took place during the birth. This grogginess can last from hours to days, especially while medication is being taken. Some women have strange dreams, or hallucinations, while coming out of general anesthesia.

Other side effects: once the endotracheal tube is removed, the woman commonly has a sore throat for a few days; a baby born by general anesthesia may have trouble nursing the first few hours, since the anesthesia may inhibit the baby's sucking instinct.

Technical Reference: *Laurence D. Colman, M.D., specializing in Obstetrics, Gynecology, Infertility, and Endocrinology, Santa Monica, California*

Sandy

Sandy was thirty-seven when her baby was born nine weeks premature. This emergency situation changed her priorities of the birth experience.

At first, I was concerned when my doctor discovered I had gestational diabetes. But then I learned it's fairly common for women, especially in their thirties or forties with their first pregnancy. The *Merck Manual* gave me more information, and I understood that as long as I followed the recommended procedures, I'd be, and my baby would be, fine. I was thankful to have a doctor who checked me for it. The diabetes had nothing to do with what was going to happen to me.

"Gestational diabetes (GDM) .... is defined as carbohydrate intolerance of variable severity with onset or first recognition during the present pregnancy.... GDM occurs in 1 to 3% of all pregnancies.

"Most women with GDM have spontaneous onset of labor at term and are delivered vaginally.... If these pregnancies are permitted to go beyond term (more than 42 weeks), the fetus is at risk for death in utero.

"Women who have had GDM should have a 2-hour oral glucose tolerance test with 75 grams of glucose at 6 to 12 weeks postpartum, to determine whether they are normal, clearly diabetic, or have impaired glucose tolerance.

"Infants of diabetic mothers require careful neonatal assessment. These infants are at risk for respiratory distress, hypoglycemia, hypocalcemia, hyper bilirubinemia, polycythemia, and hyperviscosity.

"It (GDM) usually disappears or becomes sub-clinical following the end of pregnancy.

"All pregnant women should be screened for GDM because unrecognized or untreated gestational carbohydrate intolerance is associated with increased fetal and neonatal loss, and higher neonatal and maternal morbidity."

—from ***The Merck Manual of Diagnosis and Therapy, Edition 15,*** edited by Robert Berkow. Copyright 1987 by Merck & Co, Inc. Used with permission.

87

We planned on as unmedicated a natural vaginal delivery as possible, and of course we expected a full-term baby. My husband and I took two Lamaze classes, although we were going to use the traditional labor and delivery suite. Lamaze, being an eight-week course, hadn't yet covered cesarean or premature births. With six classes to go, Carolyn was born nine weeks early. The entire experience was unlike anything we anticipated, or even thought about. We weren't even close to thinking, "What if we can't have a vaginal delivery?" "What if our baby's premature?"

Cesarean was never in our minds. Neither of my sisters needed a cesarean, and one has four children, the other has two. My mother had four children, and even though her first was in a breech position, he was born vaginally, too.

There are certain factors in a mother's makeup, the pregnancy, etcetera, that indicate the possibility of a premature delivery. That wasn't the case with me. Even at thirty-seven-years-old, I had a textbook pregnancy. Evidently what happened to me could happen to anyone.

My placenta separated for no apparent reason. I hadn't fallen or hurt myself, or done anything strenuous. I just started bleeding one day. I never had any contractions, I never had any labor; I simply did not stop bleeding. They kept thinking it was going to stop, and it didn't.

They don't know why it happened. Normally, people who have situations like mine, with the separated placenta, have high blood pressure or they smoke or are under a lot of stress. None of those things applied to me. They generally have intense labor, and I had no labor. So nothing about mine was typical, which defied everyone's understanding.

I don't think I could have been prepared for the kind of birth I had. I wouldn't have read a book about premature birth. I had absolutely no clue. There was no reason for me to read it, but perhaps I should have read about possible complications. There was no reason for me to think I was going to have a premature baby.

After fifteen hours in the hospital, lying flat on my back, being monitored, with no contractions, and her heartbeat steady as a rock, I got up. And the bleeding started again, quite profusely. Her heartbeat went up and they decided there was no point in having me lie around any longer; they were going to have to take the baby.

There really wasn't much warning because they had kept saying, "Well, the bleeding is going to stop. Everything is going to be fine. The heartbeat is steady." Then when I woke up at six in the morning, I was told, "Surgery—we're taking the baby." I was terrified!

Everything was very positive before I was informed I had to have surgery. The labor and delivery nurses were absolutely fantastic! My doctors were very good and supportive. They were totally in tune with my fears and disillusionments because my baby's birth wasn't going the way it was supposed to.

They were also concerned about getting in touch with my husband. It was almost seven o'clock in the morning, and he had been at the hospital until eleven the night before. There was something wrong with the phone at home, and I couldn't get through. I wanted him with me, and wanted him to know what was happening.

They took me into the operating room without talking to my husband. I was very upset, but fortunately he was in the recovery room when I came-to. The baby had been born, and immediately swept down to the neonatal intensive care unit.

They gave me general anesthesia for the emergency cesarean. Since it was an emergency, they had to do the incision vertically so they could get her out as quickly as possible—because they didn't know her condition. The external scar is horizontal, but the internal incision is vertical. That means if I have another baby, it will also be a cesarean. With much apology, they told me if I were to get pregnant again, I should not attempt a vaginal delivery.

The hardest part of the birth was the suddenness of it, the absolute unexpected nature of it. A nice thing was, the minute I was awake enough, before they took me to my room from the recovery room, they took me into the NICU to see our baby.

I saw this tiny creature lying on a little tray [and] being monitored, and I foolishly thought, "Oh gosh, she looks okay; she's just a real small baby." Later I learned the first thing preemies do is spend three days getting worse. That first day I thought everything was fine.

She weighed just three pounds, eight ounces, and had a severe respiratory problem which they didn't recognize until she was almost three days old. Then she was very, very sick and on a ventilator, not breathing on her own.

The day she was born, I thought to myself, "Well, our very small, pink baby is down the hall with wonderful people taking care of her."

I didn't feel any exhilaration after her birth, and I've talked to new mothers who are so elated—everything is great, and they're proud of what they've done. I didn't have any of that. I was still pretty frightened and totally unprepared for dealing with a premature baby.

Our baby was in the hospital seven weeks. It was a very long time. I was in the hospital five days. When I left, I always felt she'd make it. I never allowed myself to think she was going to die.

My husband probably entertained the notion, because he's more realistic. He'd ask, "How sick is she? What can we do about it? What can *you* do about it?" If the answer was, "We really can't do anything about it," he wanted to know that was the answer.

I never wanted to know that answer, so I was never willing to believe we could lose her. But it was quite awhile before we were convinced she was going to be fine, because she was on oxygen therapy for eleven days. At that point, I felt very positive because it had been our big concern—now she no longer needed machines to breathe for her. Carolyn could breathe on her own!

After that she had a couple of little setbacks, but mostly it was a matter of growing and getting strong enough to have something besides an IV solution. She finally got old enough to learn how to suck, to learn how to drink out of a bottle, and to learn how to nurse.

It wasn't until she had been in the hospital for six weeks that Carolyn started drinking milk. She never had anything but breast milk. I used a pump several times a day so I was ready when Carolyn was finally able to drink. She had half-strength, then three-quarters strength, then full-strength, first through a nasal tube, then from a little bottle or straight from the source.

I didn't suffer many physical problems. Carolyn was born on a Wednesday morning, and I walked down the hall to see her that first day. My doctor's orders were, "Get them out of bed."

90

I had staples in my stomach, but I also had a big incentive—the only way I was going to see my child was to get up and walk down to see her. My nurse didn't even offer me a wheelchair. She said, "Well, aren't you going to go see your daughter?" So I got up and went to see my baby.

They were very encouraging of parental involvement, especially about fathers' participation. Every time Jim walked into the unit, a nurse would say, "Well, looks like Carolyn's diapers are wet, Dad," or "Do you think Carolyn is hungry, Dad?" But they were always very ready to back off if you looked uncomfortable, if you didn't want to do it, if you were frightened of the procedure, or whatever. They were there to give help if you wanted it, and they were there to let you do it if you wanted to.

I learned I had much more to think about than the birth itself. I was more concerned about my daughter than how *I* felt. It was only on reflection that I thought, "This is really a crummy deal. I'm never going to have the birth I thought I was going to have— vaginally, with breathing, and all that stuff." The good part is I won't have to learn all those silly breathing exercises, how to push and deal with labor pain. Instead, I'll just have to recover from abdominal surgery, which is no treat either.

In the seven weeks we spent going to the hospital every day—I would go in twice, my husband once—eighty-five round trips (we had to count them for taxes), we saw a lot of younger women and men with premature babies in the same unit. One thing my husband and I commented on to each other was that being older parents seemed to have helped us through it. We went through some rough times before, not necessarily together, not necessarily concerning a child, but we've lived a bit more of life than some of the other parents. People were continually amazed at our calm attitude in a scary situation. My response was, "I don't have a choice. This is my child and she's very sick. If I'm going to see her, I'm going to get in the car and go to see her, because that's the only way I can, and I'm going to see her every day."

When things weren't going well, we just went over and hung around, and held her, and talked to her. Even before we could hold her, we'd go in and talk to her and touch her, let her know we loved her and wanted her to come home with us.

Introduction to Chapter 10
Paraplegic Mother

In the following story, a paraplegic woman shares the story of her first pregnancy and childbirth experience. Certain risks during pregnancy may affect childbirth, especially for a paraplegic woman. The most common risk is a urinary tract infection, which if not diagnosed or treated can lead to pre-term labor, and a premature baby. A paraplegic woman may not be able to feel that labor. Other common problems in pregnancy, such as constipation and surplus weight gain, are magnified in a paraplegic because of her more sedentary life.

An important thing to consider is the emotional effect of being pregnant and having a child when the mother is paralyzed. It's crucial for her to think about her self-image, her support system, and how much her husband can do to help after the birth. There's no problem with conception because of the paraplegia, and there is no reason to forego childbearing, if that's a part of a woman's general life plan. Paraplegic women should feel assured that although possible problems may occur during pregnancy, these can be anticipated and dealt with.

One recommendation is to have the woman's urine checked by a lab at least once each trimester, so that if there is an infection it can be treated. Paraplegic women are also likely to develop bed sores, particularly if they have to be on bed rest during any part of the pregnancy.

Depending on the part of the spine affected, the woman may have some feeling in her abdomen and be able to detect when she is having contractions. Someone else may have to advise her when to use the muscles required for pushing. Internal examinations should be done throughout the pregnancy, to determine any changes in softening, thinning, or dilatation of the cervix.

Because the neuropathways are interrupted, paraplegic women will feel contractions more in their abdomen, if at all, so they need to pay attention to that, to prevent pre-term labor from bringing on the birth.

The greatest risk during childbirth for paraplegic women is autonomic hyperreflexia—adrenalin causes the blood vessels to constrict, thereby accelerating the heart, and increasing the mother's blood pressure. This can be dangerous if not kept in check, since if undetected there's the risk of the mother having a stroke.

Paraplegic women can attempt a vaginal delivery, but it's probably wise for them to have an IV at the onset of labor, in case there's a need for medication.

Technical Reference: *Laurence D. Colman, M.D., specializing in Obstetrics, Gynecology, Infertility and Endocrinology, Santa Monica, California*

Patty

Patty, paraplegic since age sixteen, describes her first pregnancy and emergency cesarean at twenty-nine. She discusses what she learned as a result of this birth, and shares her plans for her second birth.

I had scoliosis as a child, and spinal fusion surgery at around thirteen. A few years following surgery, paralysis started to set in, and they weren't sure if that was due to scoliosis or something else. They just never discovered what caused the paralysis.

By sixteen, I had to be in a wheelchair because I was paraplegic—I had full use of my hands and arms, but couldn't move my legs or feet. At the time, I was so busy coping I didn't think about how it was affecting me. Life was easier for me then. It grew more difficult when I became an adult. There were times in my twenties and thirties when I was more anxious and depressed than when I was in my teens. Perhaps I had too much to deal with when I was young and put the feelings off until later. This is what I've learned in counseling, and it makes sense, because the feelings have to come out some time.

My husband, Bob, and I were married four years when our son was born. We were both in school when we got married, so we waited until our education was completed before starting our family.

I didn't know another paraplegic mother to talk to about what birth would be like. I went in unknowing and apprehensive. Being pregnant and having children were part of my plans for the future, but I was anxious about how I was going to take care of a baby in a wheelchair.

First of all, I had hopes of finding an obstetrician who specialized in, or at least knew something about, paraplegic people. The best I could do was a recommendation from my neurologist. He

95

told me about a local obstetrician, and she treated me as a regular, pregnant patient. She was new, young, and probably didn't know any better. I certainly didn't know any better either.

When I called the two rehabilitation hospitals and got nowhere, I didn't know where else to turn. I was angry, because it felt like nobody understood what I was going through.

The other thing that was hard in the hospital was [that] it was not set up for someone in a wheelchair. They didn't understand how to take care of a paraplegic person. I had to answer a lot of questions for them and that made things harder.

My pregnancy went along very nicely. When I was pregnant, I felt more like I was part of the real world, and it gave me a better body image. It was harder for me to move around and to get in and out of cars, but I worked, teaching in school, until I was five months along. Then I tutored at home until I was about six months pregnant. That was easy. I was able to meet all the demands along the way.

My water broke at seven-and-a-half months. I went into the hospital and was dilated three centimeters. I then had an emergency cesarean. I was going to have a C-section anyway, but a planned one. I had general anesthesia, because they didn't want to do a spinal block due to the prior back surgery.

Since I had general anesthesia for the surgery, I didn't see my baby immediately after birth. They gave me something which reverses the effect of the anesthesia, and I came out of it quite quickly. I wasn't in real good shape, but enough to know what happened.

My baby was about six-and-a-half weeks early, but he was a large premature baby and weighed six pounds. They were really surprised about his weight, and didn't anticipate any problems when they first observed him. He scored well on the Apgar scale—he received nine points at one minute, and nine at five minutes. The Apgar scale was developed by Dr. Virginia Apgar, a pediatrician, as a way of determining the immediate health of a newborn. There are five different categories which receive a 0, 1, or 2 rating, at one and five minute readings. All hospitals use this scale when a baby is born, and chart the results.

Two or three hours following his birth, his breathing became labored. That's typical for a preemie, to have some kind of respiratory problem, although it doesn't always show up so soon. The body gets worn out trying to keep up. He had hyaline membrane disease, and also jaundice. He was transferred to a neonatal intensive care unit, at another hospital, about four hours after birth.

He spent the first twelve days of his life in the hospital. At the time, I was so busy getting through it, I didn't consider my feelings. Looking back on it, it was horrendous. I was in a very busy maternity ward, without my baby, and I developed some sort of an infection—like a uterine infection. I was very sick, [and] my baby was sick and was taken away in an ambulance at four o'clock in the morning. It was real hard on me.

My husband went back and forth between hospitals. Luckily, they were only ten minutes apart. I was in the hospital five days, which is about normal for a cesarean delivery. Mobility-wise, and since I don't have feeling below the waist, it was probably easier for someone like me to have this kind of surgery. I was told not to drive for six weeks. But ... because I had to, I was driving to see my son in intensive care and spending the day there, when I had been out of the hospital for only two days. I felt horrible, because I was still getting over my infection—I was light-headed and breaking out in sweats. I felt I had to see my baby, so I put myself through that. I didn't have a chance to think about my own recovery, because there was too much else going on.

We were just starting our own business, and my husband was also a paramedic for L.A. City. It was such a difficult and trying time. He did everything he could to help, but when something like this happens, I don't think anyone can do enough for you.

The baby and I didn't have good bonding at first, and I think that was a problem. I didn't feel very close to him when he came home from the hospital. And also it seems like when you have a premature baby, family and friends keep their distance 'cause they're afraid to get too close and get you excited—in case something happens. I wasn't getting the blue balloon bundles and the little baby clothes. I wasn't ignored, but I wasn't given the kind of attention that makes having a baby so exciting. Everyone was really scared.

In the hospital, they said they'd know within three days whether our baby had a good chance to make it. If they get over respiratory problems quickly, they're usually fine. If they have to labor with it, then it takes them longer to recover, if at all. He was big and strong, so he did well. However, it was touch-and-go for the first few days.

I'd be lying in one hospital with a temperature of a hundred and four, calling the neonatologist at a second hospital to hear what the oxygen level was for my son. I'd do that at three o'clock and at five o'clock in the morning. I didn't sleep much either. It was really crazy. The hardest thing was [that] there wasn't anyone around to support me in what I was emotionally going through, even though we have a very large, close family.

What I learned from my experience with a preemie is, even if there's a possibility of the baby not making it, family and friends still need to give you the same support they would give if you had a healthy baby.

I used a breast pump at the hospital so I could breast-feed, which I began when he was about a week old. I developed a good milk supply by using the pump. They started him on bottles, and because the baby doesn't have to work as hard to get milk, that made it a little difficult when I started breast-feeding. Many premies have trouble breast-feeding, but he didn't. I think some of our bonding began at that time.

I didn't have any in-house help when I began taking care of Chris. It'll be different with the next baby. [Patty is three months pregnant with her second baby.] I don't know how much we were in denial about what we needed. I had my grandmothers coming over to watch the baby for a few hours at a time, but we didn't have a consistent person to help me with the baby. I pretty much did everything, since the house was all set up for me to do the things I needed to do.

There's a big difference between how we're planning for this birth, as compared with what we did for Chris's birth. Because Chris was our first, we calculated when we wanted him to be born. We knew we wanted to have two children, and were going to wait five or six years before having the second one because it would be easier that way. Then I could avoid having to take care of two babies, or a baby and a toddler at the same time.

When I became pregnant for the second time, I decided to see a perinatologist. This type of doctor has two more years of training than a regular obstetrician has. I have a lot more confidence now, to get what I need and not settle for second best. I was more naive the first time. I'm being monitored very closely for things like bladder infections, which they think may have caused the premature rupture of the amniotic sac. My previous obstetrician didn't consider bladder infections to be a problem.

This perinatologist is recommending a series of diagnostic ultrasounds, and is watching for any kind of infection. I will be more closely observed, toward the end of my pregnancy, for a bladder infection—especially because of what happened with Chris. The hospital we've chosen also has a neonatal intensive care unit. Our perinatologist practices at the hospital where Chris was when he was in intensive care. If I do have a premature baby, we'll both be at the same hospital.

I think women's intuition, even for a first baby, is sometimes greater than a doctor's. I felt like something was happening—I felt different. The obstetrician pretty much ignored it. I was even in her office the day before the birth, and she thought the contractions were Braxton Hicks contractions and were nothing to be alarmed about. She didn't even do a pelvic exam that day. This doctor is doing a pelvic exam every month, 'cause I wouldn't necessarily feel contractions and know if I'm dilating, but he'd be able to determine if my cervix is thinning out and softening.

I did feel contractions, but not the sharp pains. I could feel the tightening of the contraction. I could also feel the baby moving around during my pregnancy. If I do begin having contractions too early, I can go on an anti-contraction medication so the baby won't be born early, and I'd also be put on bed rest. There are several things that can be done to hold off having a baby, at least for several weeks. It could probably have been done with my son.

When I first went to see the perinatologist, I thought he'd give me a list of all the things I was supposed to do, and a list of things I couldn't do. It didn't turn out that way. He didn't see any reason why I'd have to be on bed rest.

Things could change toward the end of the pregnancy—some women have to be on bed rest if their first was premature. And this doctor has had some experience with paraplegic women. That makes me feel better.

Even though I am five years older with this pregnancy, I'm the same weight I was when I was pregnant with my first, and my general health is good. I'm not as apprehensive and anxious about how I'm going to take care of a newborn and then a crawling baby, because I've done that and I know now I can do [it]. Everything is at my level—the crib, the changing table, and even the playpen.

When my son was a baby, he helped out a lot. Instead of crawling at first, he learned to pull himself up on my wheelchair. Babies and children learn very quickly what their moms can and can't do. From early on, he and I had good intuitions. He knew if he hurt himself, he had to help me to get to him if he wanted to be picked up.

We made our house ultra-safe. There's no area in the house I can't get to. It worked out, even though it wasn't easy. It's not like I can have a baby on a hip and cook at the same time. All the movements have to be calculated. When the phone rang, I had to put the baby out of the way so I could get to the phone. It worked as long as I thought ahead of time what I was going to be doing.

The main reason I'm going to have help with a second baby is because my son will be going into first grade. I'll need to drop him at school and pick him up, as well as take him on errands, or … [drive him to] other activities. The help will be nice.… so I can get my son and take him to the park and spend time with him, knowing the baby is being taken care of at home.

I've already included my son in some of my prenatal doctor's visits. He's been aware of the pregnancy from the beginning. At first I wasn't sure how he'd feel about it, because he's a typical only child—very indulged with attention. He's so used to one-on-one, but he's really excited. There are many baby cousins in the family, so he knows babies aren't all fun and games, and they're not like dolls. He wanted to take care of Mommy when he first found out. He reminded me to take my prenatal vitamins and eat healthy snacks—he was really cute. Now I think he's gotten bored with the whole thing. It's been three months since I told him about the pregnancy, and I think the novelty has worn off. He talks about it occasionally and seems excited then.

The first time it took three months for me to get pregnant, and the second time was even easier and quicker than the first. I have some fears about the second birth, since I had a bad experience the first time. I just don't want to think about it a whole lot, and I know I'll do whatever I have to do when the time comes. I know I have a good doctor, so I let it go—or else it would drive me crazy. The doctor told me if the baby is small, perhaps if I'm one month early, I could try for a vaginal delivery. He told me he's ninety percent sure I'll have a C-section, which is fine with me. I don't know if I want to deal with a last minute decision, wondering if my body can handle a natural birth.

It's not always true that a paraplegic must have a cesarean, but most doctors prefer to do a C-section just so they don't have to worry about any complications due to paraplegia. I'm hoping I'll have more time to prepare for anesthesia, and be able talk to an anesthesiologist to see if he's comfortable giving me a spinal or an epidural with the condition of my back. Having an epidural would definitely be nicer, because a general just knocks me out so much. … I feel kind of depressed and anxious, and a whole number of things which aren't pleasant.

My husband is hoping this birth will be less hectic than the first one. We had been to the C-section class together, before the first birth. Taking the class allows husbands to join their wives in the delivery room. It was such a last minute thing at Chris's birth. The maternity ward was flying around getting an anesthesiologist and a pediatrician, and they told my husband he couldn't be with me. I mean of all times to say, "No."

Just four hours before, I was in bed watching the news. To hear he couldn't be with me was very upsetting. I'm rather nervous about hospitals, because I've had so much history with them. I really needed him there. He had to get persuasive, which he's [especially] good at … because of his job. He told them, "I need to be with my wife."

They said, "I'm sorry. This is an emergency. We're giving her a general. We're not comfortable with you being in the room."

He really had to stand up for himself, and at last he was allowed to be in the room with me. They weren't real happy, but we got what we wanted.

I don't think it will come up again. We'll talk to the doctor about it, and let him know how we feel if there's an emergency.

Someone in our family will take care of Chris when we have to leave for the hospital. Fortunately, they live close by. We have six grandmothers in the area, and one of them will be with Chris at the hospital, so he can come in right after the baby's born. He's at such a neat age—almost six-years-old. He won't be nervous about being away from Mommy.

101

I don't know how other handicapped women handle being a mother. What I've found is everybody's handicap is so unique, and their needs are different. What one mother may need to be able to take care of her baby would be different from what another handicapped mother needs.

I called two separate rehabilitation hospitals when I was pregnant with my first. Neither one of them had any obstetricians who could help me, or any support groups for handicapped women.

I'm not sure what kind of advice I could give, except to have good insurance, plenty of support, and have your life as organized as you can. Make sure the nursery is set up well, and if you can afford household help, use it. In hindsight, I should have had paid help. If we had a little more money, or if somebody had persuaded me to have help, I would have done it. I'm so used to being a big, brave girl. It would have helped to have had someone take care of the household things or take care of the baby, so I wasn't doing it all.

As far as doctors, that was probably the hardest thing to find. For a paraplegic person, the best thing would be to have a perinatologist, and also have the support of the other doctors you use, such as neurologists, urologists, or orthopedic doctors.

I did prepare quite a bit when I was pregnant the first time. I went to my orthopedic doctor who took a back x-ray. He wanted to make sure my spine was strong enough. I had so many questions, such as, "What about the curvature of my back? Will it be strong enough to carry a baby? Will I have the capacity?"

I learned that my spine was strong enough, and even if a mother's back is curved in a strange way, babies find their space. I was reassured by him, and my neurologist said it was fine, it wouldn't change my condition. My urologist said it was okay. I did get a lot of reassurances, but I was still scared to death. The doctors were all giving me the go ahead, but somehow I didn't find the right obstetrician.

I haven't found any paraplegic women who have had children since I've had Chris. I've been out in the world a lot, too. I went to Cal State Northridge for four years. Most paraplegic people seem to be men, for one thing. Every once in awhile I'll see a mother-looking person in a wheelchair, but not someone I can become acquainted with—like at a conference or a convention. I don't think there are a lot of them out there.

When I was pregnant with my first, I had this feeling I was diving into a deep pool, and then I'd find out if I could swim or not. I knew that's what I was doing and it was a horrible feeling. I don't think having a baby has been the hardest thing for me. When a child is four or five and ... [has] to be disciplined, that's even harder. That has nothing to do with being in a wheelchair. I think children are very challenging, and most of my apprehension is about disciplining two of them. You have to be so conscious of what you say when you have children. They change their behavior through reacting to what is said to them. I'm not as concerned about the physical aspects, as about the emotional aspects.

Even with a large family, I didn't get as much support as I thought I was going to get. I think I expected too much from them. People have their own lives and their own busy schedules, and I found myself getting a little angry that I wasn't getting more help. It wasn't their problem, it was mine. For this baby, I'll have more hired help, and only rely on family as back-up support.

Chris was an easy baby to take care of. He ate every three hours, but he slept between those times and that made things very manageable. I was still busy non-stop, with one thing or another, taking care of his physical needs. I think his most challenging age was nine months to eighteen months. Luckily, Chris intuitively knew what I needed of him. He had excellent comprehension from a very early age. I could trust him to not run into the street, for instance. He learned that if he wanted to go somewhere, he had to crawl into the car and help me with the car seat.

I'm now thirteen weeks pregnant, and we've heard the baby's heartbeat. We don't have any genetic problems on either side of our families, so [either] I'm not concerned about the baby's health or I just don't want to spend time thinking about that, too. The doctor is not requiring amniocentesis, because I'm borderline at thirty-four. The risk of having a miscarriage due to the procedure is actually greater than something being wrong with the baby. [In a woman under thirty, the chance of finding a genetic problem with the fetus is less than the chance of miscarriage. In a woman older than forty, the chance of finding a genetic abnormality is greater than the risk of miscarriage, and that is why it is recommended.] Therefore, the doctor doesn't want to have it done.

Although I was frightened about having a baby, I felt like a proud pioneer doing something unique—and we're fortunate that everything turned out so beautifully. Since my body hasn't always done what bodies usually do, being able to have a baby was extra special. And we've learned how to avoid problems for our second baby. The negatives were more than overcome by the positives—things like feeling the baby move inside me, and then holding our baby for the first time. Now we look forward to our second child.

Introduction to Chapter 11
Scheduled Cesarean

(Please also read "Introduction to Chapters 9 and 12.")

When a cesarean is scheduled, a number of procedures take place before the actual surgery begins. The woman's temperature and blood pressure are taken, and the baby's heartbeat is checked. Some of the pubic hair will be shaved to reduce the bacteria—all bacteria cannot be eliminated, but the area near the site of the incision must be as sterile as possible. Hospitals differ as to whether they shave part of the pubic hair or shave the upper abdomen and the pubic hair.

Most hospitals do not require an enema, although some may give an enema on the evening prior to the surgery. Some feel it helps the mother during surgery and during the early recovery period, when it's uncomfortable for her to move her bowels.

A catheter (a thin tube that drains urine from the bladder, into a bag on the side of the patient's bed) is used for all women who have cesareans. Exactly when the catheter is inserted varies from hospital to hospital. The actual insertion of the catheter may be mildly uncomfortable, but it can't be felt once it's in place. It takes only a few minutes for insertion, and breathing in a relaxed, slow rhythm is helpful during this short time.

The reason for the catheter is to keep the bladder empty, since it rests right over the uterus. To prevent injury to the bladder, it needs to be moved aside during surgery, and this is easier when the bladder is void and small. A catheter also eliminates the need for a bedpan or trips to the bathroom in the hours immediately following birth, and is usually removed twelve to twenty-four hours after surgery, although in some cases it's left in place for a few days.

There are two types of anesthesia considered for a C-section: general—only used for an emergency cesarean; and regional—such as an epidural.

After the surgery, nurses examine the abdomen to determine the height of the uterus. They press on the abdomen to put pressure on the top part of the uterus (fundus) to push the accumulated blood out through the vagina and encourage the uterus to contract.

105

The patient can do specific exercises to help restore her emotional and physical well-being. She can begin walking as early as the first day after surgery. It will feel like her insides are going to fall out, but she can be assured that won't happen. As long as she takes medication, she'll be able to move with little pain and be on the road to a speedy recovery.

Technical References: *American Baby Guide To Parenting, Gallery Books, 1989; Pregnancy & Childbirth: The Complete Guide For A New Life, Tracy Hotchner, Avon Books, 1979*

Sally

A planned cesarean birth was scheduled for Sally, due to her baby being in a breech (feet down) position. Sally's sister was a tremendous support, and coached her through the entire procedure. In this story, the benefits of knowing ahead of time what to expect during birth are emphasized.

I hardly showed when I was pregnant, because my baby was in a breech position and I'm really long-waisted. People thought she was going to be really tiny. But she wasn't at all—she was just standing up. She weighed seven pounds, six ounces, and was twenty-one-and-a-half inches long. My friends thought she stayed in a breech position because I have a tipped uterus.

It was a fairly stressful pregnancy, mainly due to my husband's and my separation when I was six months pregnant, and the emotional problems caused by that—before and after the separation. Until I was about seven months pregnant, I thought I was going to have a normal, natural birth. I wasn't afraid at all. I've wanted a baby since I was five-years-old.

By the beginning of my eighth month, my doctor thought the chances of having a vaginal delivery were quite slim—so, a month before the due date, I pretty much knew I was going to have a cesarean. A date was set for surgery. I was happy—I was relieved, because I had real fears about labor and how I'd cope with the pain.

I chose to have my baby in a hospital because I wanted to have a doctor at the birth. I wasn't thinking of having a midwife or a home birth. When I heard I was going to have a cesarean, I knew there wouldn't be any pain and that sounded good.

I felt prepared for my birth experience, largely due to having a very good Lamaze instructor. We learned about what to expect in the hospital; what kinds of medications were available, and what side-effects they had on mother and baby. We also learned breathing techniques for different stages of labor, and different positions to try during birth. She informed us about the most current information related to childbirth and parenting. Included in the course was one evening on cesarean birth, and at that time I knew I was going to have one, so I really tuned in to it. I read many books on pregnancy and childbirth, too.

A lot of people told me, "Don't let them insist on a cesarean. You can have the baby turned." [But] I decided, if she's breech, I'm not going to have doctors turning her.... I had heard horror stories about that, too. I always thought it was interesting how pregnant women hear so many negative things, especially when they're in their most vulnerable state. Fortunately, I had a lot of confidence and trust in my doctor, who took the time to explain procedures and back up information with examples.

To be ready for birth, I attended prenatal exercise classes and Lamaze classes, and both were quite helpful. I prepared my breasts for breast-feeding by toughening them up with dry washcloths, and didn't have any problems when I began nursing in the hospital.

My water broke a week before the C-section was scheduled. I went the hospital, after speaking to my doctor. It wasn't an emergency, or they would have knocked me out and taken the baby within three minutes. Once there, I called everybody and said, "Okay, the schedule is changed. I'm going to have the cesarean now. She's arriving a week early."

But right before the surgery I was afraid. In the back of my mind, I guess I was most scared of dying on the table and not knowing if my baby was going to be healthy.

My older sister had an emergency cesarean. She went through about twelve hours of labor, and then they finally realized her baby was in distress. The umbilical cord was wrapped around her neck, so they got the baby out as quickly as possible. In my mother's family, all of the women had vaginal deliveries. Only my sister and I had surgical deliveries.

What stands out most about the cesarean is that it was so positive. Women shouldn't be afraid of it, as long as they have competent doctors and nurses. Since I was so fearful of the pain of natural childbirth and delivery, it was actually a relief to me to have my baby born in this manner.

My sister coached me through surgery—she was a tremendous support person. The reason she was able to be so helpful was due to her personal experience with cesarean birth—although she had general anesthesia and was asleep during the delivery.

For my cesarean, I had an epidural. I was glad to be awake and alert while the surgery took place—it helped me feel like I was more connected to the birth process. There was this great anesthesiologist who had a good sense of humor. Everybody was laughing—there was a light-hearted feeling. We practically had a party in the operating room.

An epidural anesthetic is a local anesthetic, injected into the epidural area of the spine, numbing all sensation from the waist down. It takes skill to administer an epidural, since the needle must be placed between the third and fourth lumbar vertebrae.

Before the anesthesia is given, the patient is required to sign a consent form as part of hospital procedures. It's also necessary for the woman to curl into a tight ball so her chin is right down on her chest—this position separates the vertebrae of the spine, and allows the anesthesiologist to pinpoint the placement of the needle. The area is numbed with a local anesthetic before the needle and catheter are carefully inserted.

Then a catheter is passed through a needle into the epidural space around the spinal cord. The needle is then removed. The anesthetic is injected through a plastic, catheter tube, which is secured to the woman's back with adhesive tape. One injection lasts about two hours, with additional doses added through the catheter as labor progresses and additional anesthesia is needed. No other pain relief is generally necessary.

The woman needs an intravenous tube placed in her arm when she has an epidural. Through the tube, glucose water and salt are given to keep her hydrated. The baby's heart rate is continuously observed by the electronic fetal heart monitor. And the mother's blood pressure is continuously watched, because there's a tendency for it to drop during epidural anesthesia. Using all this equipment means the mother has to stay in bed for most of her labor. She'll have to consider that, and determine how she'll spend her labor, before the epidural is given.

Additional risks of using epidural anesthesia are: if the epidural is administered before five centimeters dilation, contractions can stop; it can cause a drop in maternal blood pressure, reducing the amount of oxygen her fetus receives; a risk of puncturing the membrane surrounding the spinal cord, which often results in a spinal headache; the epidural takes ten to twenty minutes to take effect; and the possibility of having a postpartum sore back.

The advantages of using an epidural are: minimal side effects to the baby, especially when Marcaine is used as the epidural; less medication is required, and it takes effect more quickly; less risk of infection—it doesn't cross the placenta, and doesn't enter the maternal bloodstream.

—**Laurence D. Colman, M.D.,** Santa Monica, California

Of course, I didn't have to worry about going into labor since I was having a C-section, and I wasn't concerned about another epidural risk—a greater chance of forceps delivery. Since the anesthetic has a relaxing effect on a woman's pelvic floor, the baby's head may not rotate into a good position for delivery, and forceps or a vacuum extractor could be employed.

I was confident an epidural was right for me. Up until the actual surgery began, I was anxious and afraid—knowing it was major surgery, and that my baby was on the way. I felt nauseous, and remember being uncomfortable. The doctors were pulling, and I was thinking I was going to throw up. I never did, but it was terrible nausea for only about two minutes. They had warned me about the nausea before it happened.

The anesthesiologist said, "Now at this point you're going to experience nausea. It's only going to last a couple [of] minutes." I remember him patting my head, and my sister was holding my hand. Once the feeling passed, I was fine, and the procedure went ahead without any problems.

When the surgery was completed and she was born, it was the most wonderful experience—better than I imagined it would be! I could cry now when I talk about it. Part of my joy was seeing that she was a girl.... I wanted a girl more than anything in the world!

My sister and I said to the doctors and nurses, before the baby was born, "We're hoping for a little vagina to come out."

When she came out, the doctor said, "It's a little vagina!"

I screamed, I was so happy! This experience brought my sister and me closer than we ever were before I had my daughter. My whole family was there after the birth, to celebrate with me.

It made such a difference to have my sister with me—she was absolutely marvelous! She had wanted a vaginal birth for herself, and wanted that for me. Of course, she was disappointed when she knew I'd have a cesarean. But mine was different, especially because it was a planned cesarean and my sister's was unexpected.

My sister's husband is a lawyer, and I think that scares doctors. The minute her baby's heart rate started to drop, the doctor went into conference with a couple of other doctors. They weren't all convinced that a cesarean was necessary, but her doctor didn't want to be sued if something happened.

My sister was really upset about not being able to have a vaginal delivery, but she has her baby and that's what's important. She went through many hours of labor which made it more difficult for her—the fact that she was so close to having a vaginal birth.

The feelings I had after the cesarean were elation—there wasn't any disappointment. When I knew I was going to have the surgery, I was kind of hoping that wouldn't change. I didn't want her to turn, because I was expecting surgery. I would have been more disheartened had she turned, and I would have had a vaginal birth—that would have been harder for me.

The cesarean was painless.... I'd like other women to know they needn't be afraid of it, or disconcerted, if they have to have one. I had a nice, healthy baby as a result, and was walking the day after surgery. I wouldn't encourage women to have a cesarean if they can prevent it, but if they have to have one it doesn't have to be a regrettable time. It was so positive for me, and not having pain was very pleasant. I could have had another baby right after she was born!

When I'm ready to have a second child, I can request to have another cesarean. I don't know if I'd schedule a repeat cesarean or choose to go into labor. I don't know what the chances are for my having another breech baby. In any case, I don't think of myself as a brave person, and I'll need to be brave in anticipation of the pain I'll most likely go through if I have a vaginal birth.

Having a baby was the most incredible thing that ever happened to me! I enjoyed my pregnancy, and her birth was very positive. My daughter has brought me more happiness than I ever dreamed of. I've been lucky in that regard. I had a lousy husband, but she more than made up for it. My family and friends helped me through my pregnancy. I had tremendous encouragement from everyone. It made a difficult time that much easier. The birth went as well as it did because I had such great support from my sister. She cut the umbilical cord and placed the baby on my chest. Then right afterward, my mom, my other sister, and my brother came in to see me and my brand new daughter. Having my family near me during this momentous occasion made the event very special for me. And as it turned out, everything that happened during the birth, I expected.

Introduction to Chapter 12
Unscheduled Cesarean

(Please also read "Introduction to Chapters 9 and 11.")

The difference between "scheduled," "unscheduled," and "emergency" cesareans, is that—"scheduled" has a date set for the surgery, and even if that date is changed the surgery is still anticipated, and merely re-scheduled. "Unscheduled" is when a vaginal delivery is planned and anticipated, but **during labor** a problem arises requiring "unscheduled" surgery. "Emergency" is when, either before or during labor, **serious** complications occur that require **immediate** surgery.

In the following story, a woman plans and anticipates a vaginal birth, but then requires an unplanned cesarean due to a projected cord prolapse (the umbilical cord preceding the baby) if she continues with labor. No one expects to have a complication occur at childbirth, such as a cord prolapse, placenta previa (the placenta blocks the baby's exit from the uterus, and will be delivered before the baby), or placenta abruptio (the placenta separates from the uterus, as in Chapter 9). These are rare occurrences, but they usually can't be predicted ahead of time.

It's important to know what kinds of complications can occur, and who to call for help if it's necessary. One suggestion is to have emergency numbers next to your phone, and also have a card with those numbers in your purse at all times. A neighbor's phone should be one of those numbers, as well as a taxi service, the nearest emergency room facility, your husband's work number, etc. It's better to be prepared for everything, with the hope it won't be needed.

The woman in the following story wasn't informed about the procedures during a cesarean section. Not knowing what was happening created more anxiety and fear for the woman and her husband. Knowledge goes a long way to help reduce a couple's fears. Some people feel if a woman prepares for a cesarean by attending a cesarean preparation class, she is more likely to have one. I think it's better to prepare for the possibility of surgery than to be surprised when it happens and feel totally unprepared and overwhelmed during the experience.

If a couple is planning a hospital birth, it's a good idea to attend a cesarean preparation class in the hospital where the birth will take place. During the class, a tour of the maternity ward is usually included. The couple will see the labor, operating, and recovery rooms, and will view slides or a video outlining the steps of the cesarean. Ask questions and be sure to get the answers you need. The information may or may not come in handy at a later time, but it's better to know what might happen than be in the dark about it.

Technical Reference: *Laurence D. Colman, M.D., specializing in Obstetrics, Gynecology, Infertility, and Endocrinology, Santa Monica, California*

Cindy

Cindy was married at thirty-eight, and within a year, had her first baby. Her attitude and philosophy helped her through the unexpected cesarean.

The kind of birth I planned was a vaginal birth, as "au naturel" as I could get. However, I was open to anything that needed to be done. I hoped to be able to do it as naturally as possible, but I didn't care if it didn't work out that way—except I definitely expected a vaginal birth.

Two weeks before my baby was due, she turned breech. Apparently, she was head down until that point. The doctor and I talked about it, and we decided to wait and see if she would turn around on her own. We opted to forego any manipulation, because I was thirty-eight and they didn't want to fool around with me. My doctor is very conservative and felt, if he had to, he'd rather do a cesarean than try version (a procedure which relaxes the uterus, and the doctor attempts to turn the baby to a head-down position by manipulating the outside of the abdomen).

We waited three weeks, a week after the due date, and she still hadn't turned. I went in for my weekly exam and was told I was three centimeters dilated. They told me I couldn't go into labor because the umbilical cord was beginning to drop down.... If I went into labor, it could prolapse [the cord would come out before the baby] causing serious complications. They would have to do a cesarean section either immediately or later that day.

I said, "Get this baby out, now!"

That was about eleven o'clock in the morning. I went to the hospital by myself—my husband Mark was at work and didn't know about any of this. They hooked me up to a monitor and called him. We waited about two hours for him to come, but he was stuck on

115

the freeway. They finally couldn't wait any longer, since the delivery room was reserved later. Just then my husband appeared.

For those two hours, I was nervous. Nobody told me what was happening. They just stuck me into one of the birthing rooms, and my sister came and sat with me. Another ultrasound scanning was done to see if the baby was still breech (as if she was going to turn around in an hour!). Mostly I just sat there.

When they decided to put me into the delivery room, they got me all prepped and then the catheter wouldn't go in. No one explained what was going on. All I knew was that it was really painful. It was traumatic ... [when] they had to put in another catheter. The first one was inserted into my vagina instead of my urethra. The doctor had to place the second one in, because the nurse couldn't seem to do it. I was very tense through that experience.

Then they hooked me up to the IV, and flooded me with the sugar water. Suddenly I started shivering, and it was uncontrollable. Even when I tried to relax, my body continued quivering. I asked the assistant obstetrician what was happening.

He told me, "The glucose and water are given to protect your blood pressure from falling too low when the anesthesia is injected, and it's common for the body to shake during this procedure." The assistant obstetrician was my saviour. Without him I don't know what I would have done. He held my hand when they gave me the epidural anesthesia. He really alleviated my fears.

My regular obstetrician came in after they set up the sterile field. With those drapes all around me, I couldn't see. When the doctor began to cut, I felt all this tugging and asked, "What are they doing?"

Again nobody told me. There was a lot of pulling and tugging. I remember talking to the anesthesiologist the entire time, saying how scared I was. He was trying to calm me down. I don't know whether they gave me morphine or what, but I was just not my normal self.

In any event, my baby was perfectly healthy. When she came out, she was absolutely gorgeous. They placed her right next to me after she was wiped off. I was crying so hard; I was so moved by it. After I saw she was perfect, it was like I didn't care about myself, and that really changed my attitude.

Before she was born, I wanted to have a vaginal birth, but that was for *me* and for my own sense of power and womanhood. When I heard her and held her and knew *this was another life,* I said, "Who cares if it's a cesarean or not? As long as my baby's okay, who cares?" That has made a very deep impression on me ever since. I hope to get pregnant again, and I don't care if it's a VBAC (vaginal birth after cesarean) or a cesarean.

My fears before the birth were basically whether I could deal with the labor. I had a ninety-nine percent feeling that everything was going to be all right. I felt healthy, [and] I had a beautiful pregnancy. I think my only fear was that I wouldn't be able to handle the labor. When I didn't have to go through it, it was irrelevant.

I took prenatal exercise classes all the way along—that was my physical preparation. My mental preparation was reading everything I could get my hands on concerning what was happening inside of me. And since I ate really well, and don't drink, smoke, or use drugs, I felt very good. I did a lot of needlepoint, and I was lucky because I didn't have to work the last half of my pregnancy. So, I was really able to enjoy the feelings. I was absolutely enthralled by being pregnant! It wasn't planned. It was a complete surprise, and I was very interested in learning about my pregnancy.

I expected labor to be so painful, from the way I heard it described, that I seriously didn't know if I was mentally strong enough to cope with it. That's all I can say. I didn't get a chance to find out what the pain would have been like since I didn't have any labor to speak of.

They tell you that motherhood is going to be one of the most memorable highlights of your life, but nothing prepares you for how powerful it is when you see that baby—at least for me. I don't think anyone can describe what it's like when you see a baby that came out of your body. I'm a changed person because of it. It's like being a member of a club that you never knew existed.

The thing that surprised me the most about the operation was that I didn't know what was going on, and I wished I had been told about each procedure every step of the way. I was at the mercy of everyone around me. I had no sense of participation—I was just someone there who was being operated on and being cut open.

117

My husband was so scared he couldn't help me. Not that he didn't want to, but ... he was overwhelmed by it. I was terribly frightened, lonely, and vulnerable.

My mother had six children, and she told me I'd forget the pain of childbirth when I saw my baby. For me, the most positive thing is that I'm a mother, and I thank God every day that I got to experience it, 'cause I'm older, and we didn't think it was in the cards for us to be parents. Then I became pregnant two months after we were married.

When I went back to see my obstetrician after our baby was born, I told him I was a terrible patient because I was hysterical and so scared. He said, "Don't feel badly about your response to the situation. It was understandable, considering what was happening to you."

No matter what, I couldn't be more happy with the result. However, I think doctors should be more sensitive to what their patients are feeling at the time, and not be afraid to tell women what's going on during childbirth. If they had a hard time getting my baby out, I wouldn't sue them for malpractice, but I'm sure they're afraid most women would.

I would have liked more openness. That would have meant that doctor and patient would have been working together, whereas, I felt he was hiding what he was doing—that I was being excluded. Here I was in perfect health and, with the exception of an appendectomy ... never in a hospital.

Everyone I know who had seen my life pattern for the last several years said, "If anyone's going to have a baby without drugs, you're the most likely candidate. And it's going to be a vaginal birth, and you'll probably deliver in an hour."

Cesarean birth just never entered my mind. My life has always been healthy and the pregnancy was uneventful and beautiful. I really hadn't focused on how the birth would be.

What I learned as a result of my birth experience is [that] I don't matter as much as I thought I did. I'm important enough to be told what's going on during childbirth, but *how* it happens is not as important as I thought it would be. As long as everybody's healthy, that's all that matters. I really felt my doctors did the right thing for me in my particular situation. It wasn't something that anybody knew about or could plan. Just as long as the baby is okay, the end justifies the means.

I've learned doctors aren't perfect. I think they take their craft too lightly. I asked one obstetrician why he went into obstetrics, and he said, "Because it's not a depressing field. There's a lot of happiness in this specialty that you might not find in geriatrics or oncology."

I still think, after awhile it just becomes a job. And it's something we just have to live with.

Another thing I've learned is not to give advice to expectant couples unless they ask for it. If they want to know what it's like to have a cesarean, I'll tell them everything that happened to me. I'll give them information, and let them deal with it.

I have a girlfriend I've known for twenty-five years, who went through the exact situation I did, thirteen months before me. She didn't tell me about the shivering and the catheter. If our situations had been reversed, and knowing her as I do, I would have told her about those occurrences. She and I had parallel experiences all the way down. If your doctor won't tell you, at least it would help to have your friends tell you about their childbirths. But I guess I never asked her.

Three years later, Cindy's second child was born vaginally, without any medication. She was happy to have had a VBAC, but it didn't matter much to her in the end. In fact, once she had the second child, she realized how meaningful both births were.

Part III

BIRTH CENTER BIRTH

Introduction to Chapter 13

First and Second Births
in a Birth Center

*When a woman arrives at the birth center, in labor, she goes to one
of the available private labor and delivery rooms and either puts on
her own gown or one belonging to the center. Her blood pressure and
temperature are checked every hour, to see that neither is raised ab-
normally. Elevated blood pressure may signify toxemia, and elevated
temperature may signify infection.*

*A midwife listens to the fetal heartbeat every twenty to thirty
minutes, with a fetoscope or a doptone (no fetal heart monitors—
machines that display the mother's and fetus' heartbeats— are used).*

*The expectant mother has more freedom of movement in a birth
center than in a hospital, because she can eat, drink, and walk about
during her labor. No medication is available, although she can relieve
labor pains by immersing herself or sitting in a large, round bathtub
filled with warm water. This tub is sometimes where the birth takes
place. A midwife is always with the patient, to attend to her needs.*

*There's no limit on the number of family and friends observing
and/or helping with the birth. For the delivery, the new mother can be
standing, sitting, squatting, lying down, or choose the position in which
she feels most comfortable.*

*An episiotomy (incision between the vagina and the anus, to avoid
possible tearing in that area during birth) is performed only five percent
of the time, whereas in hospitals it's done for over ninety percent of
births. The reason for such a low percentage in a birth center is due
to the use of hot packs on the woman's buttocks, massaging olive oil
on the perinium (the posterior area of the vagina), and not rushing the
delivery.*

*There are several reasons a woman would have to be transferred
from a birth center to a hospital: she developed an infection during
labor, revealed in her elevated body temperature; excessive bleeding
during labor—measured by the amount absorbed on the bed sheet. If,
within a half-hour, the blood spot is larger than a fifty-cent-piece, she
is taken to a hospital; meconium (the baby's first bowel movement)*

123

released is not transparent; the fetus is in a breech (not head-down) position.

Technical Reference: *Nancy McNeese, Certified Nurse Midwife and owner of the Natural Childbirth Institute & Women's Health Center, in Culver City, California*

Kerry

Kerry is the mother of two children, both born in a birth center run by certified nurse midwives. She proved to herself, twice, that she was able to give birth without medication.

The one thing I was convinced of was that it was possible to have babies without being drugged. In spite of all the stories I'd read and the people I'd talked to, I knew it had to be possible. For so many years there were no drugs. Maybe somebody's doing something wrong that requires the drugging of women. Maybe if women knew what they needed to do they could avoid that.

I had the normal fears everyone has during pregnancy, hoping the baby would be fine, yet afraid something would go wrong. Not so much the birth, but that the baby wouldn't be perfect.

To prepare for the birth, my husband and I went to childbirth classes, and I read everything I could get my hands on for years and years. I was thirty-one, and I'm not really sure why, but the subject of childbirth fascinated me.

Even with all the classes and the reading, we weren't prepared for our first baby's actual birth. It started slowly. I went from Sunday night until Tuesday night having contractions constantly, but I slept through them and ate through them. I went on with my life for two days, and then the contractions speeded up. I got to the point where I felt I couldn't deal with them.

Then when I started pushing, her heart rate wasn't coming up. They had me alternate positions. I started out on my left side, changed to my right side, and then went to my hands and knees. Then I squatted, and her heartbeat came up. With each position change, Michael had to support me. He had his arms under my arms, holding me for forty-five minutes while I pushed. He never gave out; he was really there for me. I don't know how I would have been able to do it without him.

125

The hardest part of my births was pushing. With Shoshana, even though it wasn't painful, it was so draining to push. With Joshua, it just hurt. Compared to a lot of my friends, I didn't have to push long, but it seemed like an eternity both times, for different reasons.

I was able to relax through everything, but I took a lot of showers. I took tons of showers! That's really all I needed to do; it was just so easy.

After sixty hours of labor, she was born at two-thirty Wednesday afternoon. Although it was extremely long, the labor was very easy because it was so gradual. I consider my labor and birth with her essentially painless.

If my births had been the other way around, I might have thought twice about having another baby because the second one was completely different.

In some ways it started out the same—fairly slowly. I woke up Saturday morning, and lost my mucous plug. I told my husband, "Don't get all excited, I could go for days." He was already crazy during the week before, so I said, "Just relax."

I was having contractions all day long, but I went out and did some things. Friends asked us for dinner that night. The wife said, "I'll invite you for dinner, hoping you won't make it, because you'll be having the baby."

We went there and as we were sitting down to dinner I thought, "These are getting a lot stronger."

I called and talked to the midwife and said, "They're really intense now. I think this is it, but I think it's going to be awhile. We're sitting down to dinner."

She said, "Okay, eat and do whatever you feel like doing."

So we finished dinner and were going to call my parents to drive over to take care of our daughter, Shoshana, while we were at the birth center.

Our friend kept saying, "I think you better call your mother."

I said, "It's all right, I have a long time."

She said, "No, you'd better call."

Another friend said, "Why don't you call, so they'll be here and you won't have to worry about it?"

I did, and my parents said they'd be at our house in an hour-and-a-half. So we had our dessert and then went home.

We arrived about ten-fifteen, and the pains were progressively stronger. My husband, Michael, stood at the door waiting for my folks, wondering if they were going to make it in time.

He said, "When your mom and dad get here, I think we should go." I still wasn't convinced, but they came, and we packed the car and got to the birth center at midnight.

I was already four centimeters dilated, and then my water broke. The midwife said, "I think things will move pretty fast now. If you want, you can get in the hot tub."

This labor was more difficult, because the contractions were much stronger. But spending time in the hot tub, when they were really intense, helped a lot. It was great in the water. When the contractions would start, I could rise up on one hand, and sort of float so there was no pressure on my spine. I was in the water about forty-five minutes when I couldn't take it anymore. I said, "I'm getting too hot. I need to get out." The contractions were getting intense and I thought, "There's no way I'm going to make it through this, because these are getting too strong!"

I got out of the tub wondering how I was going to survive. I felt like I had to push. I started pushing at one o'clock, and Joshua was born a half-hour later.

The quickness of the labor surprised me. I didn't expect it. After going so long with Shoshana, I figured the second baby would be faster, but I didn't expect it to be that much faster!

I honestly don't know what helped to speed up my second delivery. I didn't use imagery. I was just able to relax, probably because in my first labor when I tensed up it hurt, so I thought, "I have to relax." And I did.

The most surprising part of my labors was the intensity of the feelings. You know, painful or not, it's an incredibly intense experience. When I started to push with Shoshana, it was like I had no control over my body, just a force making me do it. After every contraction, I thought, "Oh, God, I can't do this anymore. I'm going to stop." Then I'd have another one, and I couldn't stop. It's amazing how engulfed in it I was—emotionally, mentally, physically, and spiritually.

There were many reasons why I had such positive experiences with my births. First of all, the birth center is wonderful—being able to go to a familiar place, where I went for all my prenatal visits. I felt the people really cared *for* me, in addition to taking care *of* me. Secondly, my mother and mother-in-law were there for both births, and of course my husband was a big part of it. It was a loving atmosphere for having a baby.

I was thinking about having a home birth even for our first baby. My husband wouldn't allow me to have a home birth. He said, "There's no way; it's not even up for discussion." I think part of me was scared of it, too, especially the first time—not knowing what it was going to be like. Even though I believe the vast majority of births are normal, I worried about what would happen if I were in that tiny percentage where things don't go normally.

The birth attendants were important to the success of my births. When Shoshana was born, there were nurses at the center, in addition to the midwives. Now there are only midwives. Tracy is a wonderful labor nurse. When I was pushing, she put cold compresses on my back or on my forehead. Without my asking, she'd say, "Are you thirsty? Do you want something to drink?" She'd hold the glass up for me. They're really sensitive to what's needed.

I also liked the fact that one person stayed with me throughout the birth. The first time, Tracy was with us from the beginning until almost the end. Nancy was there for the last couple of hours. This time I got Nancy, the midwife, from beginning to end, because no matter how long the birth takes the same midwife is with you.

My husband gave me tremendous emotional support— knowing he was there, and cared, and was willing to do whatever I wanted him to do. With Shoshana, I didn't have back labor, but he put pressure on my lower back for a long time, just because it felt better.

From my birthing experiences, I gained respect for every other woman who has given birth. I learned you can give birth without drugs. It was nice to prove my thesis. It's encouraging [to know] that even though, generally, chemical intervention is given for labor and birth these days, it's possible to give birth without all that. I know people who've had really long, painful labors, and are still able to do it without intervention. We're capable of much more than we think we are.

To prepare women more for what the experience of labor is like, I would tell women that it is like being in an altered state. I don't know if withdrawal is the right word, but I seemed to go inside myself, and nothing existed beyond two feet around me. I was completely oblivious to everything unless it immediately impacted upon me. That was real surprising, because I didn't expect it. It was such an all-consuming event that there was nothing else. There was no time and there was no world outside of me. When I had to, I could go out, but just for the short moments, and then I would retreat back in.

Another interesting aspect was my spiritual connection to the babies I was carrying. I had recently converted to Judaism. I was only a month pregnant, and I was aware when I went through the process, that it was not only for me, but for me and whoever was within me. I was conscious each time I was pregnant that I was bringing a new Jewish person into this world, and that was exciting for me. Having newly come to it myself, it was like I was already increasing it. That was really wonderful!

Choosing names for our daughter was very difficult for us. We knew it was going to be an "S" name for Michael's father. It's funny because the whole time I was pregnant with her, I knew it was a girl. About halfway through, we came up with Shoshana. We started out choosing Serai, if it was a girl, but the more we said it, we thought it was a pretty name but not quite right. Then we found Shoshana. We didn't decide on a boy's name until a week before her birth, when we ended up with Seth, which is not my favorite name. So I prayed, "Please let me be right. Let it be a girl!"

The second time, the names came fairly easily. The girl's name was Tova. We were looking for a "T" name, after my grandfather. When we couldn't agree on a "T" name for a boy, we decided to use one for the middle, and we both loved Joshua Tov. Even though I felt I wasn't going to have a boy, I thought, "It doesn't matter, either sex is fine." The first time, it made a big difference to me whether it was a boy or a girl, because I didn't want the boy's name, not because I didn't want a boy.

When Shoshana was born, my mother said, "It's a girl!"

I never even looked at her, I just put my arms around her after Nancy laid her on my chest. She said, "Aren't you going to look and see if it's a girl?" I looked, but it was superfluous because I knew she was. The second time, I helped to lift Joshua out, so I was probably the first to see he was a boy.

Up until the actual first birth, I wasn't sure how I was going to feel about it, but I especially enjoyed having my mother there. It was nice because she doesn't remember much about her births. She had spinals for both of them, and also had miserable experiences being left alone during her labors. I thought she'd like being at my child's birth, and it turned out she did. She thought it was wonderful!

The second time, she said she didn't want to be in on it because it was emotionally overpowering. She said, "I'm glad I was there for Shoshana's birth, but it was just too emotional for me." It brought back feelings she had. She said, "I'll be there with you, but I'm just not going to be in the room."

I said I totally understood and we asked her to go with us, to take care of Shoshana. Then, as it turned out, she came in the room for the birth because she heard Michael go get his mother, and thought, "He's not going to get me, and I want to be there."

Only three-years-old, Shoshana was asleep, but right after the birth my mother woke her and brought her into the room. We have pictures of her staring at Joshua, and watching carefully while Michael cut the cord. She saw them stitch me up, and she was fascinated by the whole thing.

God, I could have kids forever. I mean, not the giving birth, but I love having kids. I always knew I wanted a family, but it amazes me how wonderful it is, how rewarding, and how frustrating sometimes.

Leboyer Birth

"Leboyer birth" is named for obstetrician Frederick Leboyer, *who wrote the book,* **Birth Without Violence,** *in 1974. It's method of delivery is intended to reduce birth trauma by creating a gentle transition from the womb to the world—dimming the lights, allowing only soft voices, and giving the newborn a warm bath—usually by the father, and perhaps with the aid of the attending physician.*

Leboyer had delivered thousands of babies, and he noticed their responses to the birth process. They were held upside down after delivery, and spanked on the bottom to start their lungs. Today they're no longer spanked, but the mucous is suctioned out of their mouths with a small aspirator. Babies lost body heat very quickly, because they were separated from their mothers and then placed in incubators, which increased their isolation. Now, skin-to-skin contact between baby and parents is encouraged immediately following childbirth.

One of the things that's emphasized today, in most birth settings, is talking softly, so the baby comes into the world in a gentler way than with loud voices or yelling—a shocking way to start life outside the womb. The ideal environment is a home setting in which a dimly-lit room provides just enough light for delivery.

This type of birth is synonymous with minimal intervention, such as avoiding an episiotomy and medications. Immediately after birth, the baby is placed on the mother's abdomen to rest and bond with her. The umbilical cord is allowed to stop pulsing before it is cut—fathers often have the privilege of cutting the cord.

Once the baby seems relaxed, the doctor assists the father in placing the baby in a tub of water, heated to body temperature. The tub is usually placed on a counter, and this is a wonderful opportunity for the dad to hold and bond with his baby, while mom rests and delivers the placenta. When the bath is over, the baby is offered mother's breast, and nurses for as long as possible.

Women who purposely want to provide their baby with a Leboyer birth, believe as Dr. Leboyer did that this gentle experience can help a little one coming into the world feel cared for and respected.

Technical Reference: *Salee Berman, C.N.M., Culver City, California*

Rose

Rose and her husband planned a Leboyer birth to minimize the trauma of a baby entering a new environment of cold air, noise, and confusion. Instead, a calm atmosphere for birth was created, including the new father bonding to his daughter when he gave her a special bath, immediately following delivery.

I had always wanted to have a very healthy birth. I didn't want medications or unnecessary interference by the medical profession. Women often had a lot more interventions, supposedly for their safety, than was vital to the baby or the mother. For our child, we wanted the best possible setting, which was safe, with the least amount of intervention.

I read about home births, midwives, birth centers, and hospitals. Taking into account my age then, twenty-nine, I realized it would probably be safer if I had a medical doctor instead of a midwife. I chose a birth center that had the most comfortable setting, with very congenial medical personnel. I liked the obstetrician very much—he was always warm and friendly. He let me plan my birth the way I wanted to have it.

My pregnancy progressed normally, so I felt fully confident I'd be able to have a natural vaginal delivery. Somewhere I read and also heard, that if you used warm vitamin E oil around the vaginal opening during the last couple months of pregnancy, the tissue would become more elastic, and there'd be less chance of needing an episiotomy. I wanted to avoid that discomfort, so I used the vitamin E oil every night. As it turned out ... [this technique] was ... successful ... when I had Elisabeth.

Everything was set for a delivery some time in mid-September. I remember my doctor said, "Please don't deliver on Rosh Hashanah, because I've missed Rosh Hashanah for the past three years now. Patients insist on delivering during that time." I made a promise it wouldn't happen then, but of course I didn't have any control over when labor would start.

At about two in the morning on September 13, I woke up to labor. I wouldn't be able to keep my promise ... it was Rosh Hashanah.

I also realized I hadn't finished making the sheets for the baby's crib. I got up very quietly so I wouldn't wake my husband, and dashed into the sewing room. Between contractions, I sewed like a mad woman, trying to get the sheets done. I remembered all the things about "pant-and-blow-breathing," and it seemed like a piece of cake—it was easy!

I called the doctor to tell him how far apart the contractions were, and he told me to come to the birth center around ten, unless my contractions got closer, sooner. I called my friend who taught childbirth classes, and she came over to assist me. By the time she arrived, I was beginning to feel spacey, and I realized my husband was feeling kind of out of it—we weren't working well as a team. ... He was sort of lost. My friend tried to show him what he could do to help me during the contractions.

After a short time, the three of us left together for the birth center. I spent the rest of the day there. I had back labor, which was very uncomfortable and quite intense. I tried lots of different positions to see whether I could find one that was more comfortable than another. Standing up made me feel nervous, because I was afraid I was going to fall over when I was concentrating on relaxing during the contractions. I still don't know how women can get through a contraction standing.

Lying on my side on the bed was more comfortable. The birth room was nicely lit—very soft, indirect lighting. We had a twin bed and there were pretty pictures on the walls—which were a pale peach color, not white. It felt very homey. The instrument table and the scale were behind a curtain, so the impression of the birth room was of a bedroom rather than a delivery room.

Finally the doctor broke my bag of water to make labor less painful—it felt like I was trying to deliver a watermelon sideways. After the water broke, it was much easier. The contractions speeded up, and before too much longer Elisabeth was crowning. I was very glad I used the oil, because my skin was stretching slowly.

I was able to deliver without any tear, and she came out without much molding of her head.

She was very quiet—she didn't cry when she came out. The doctor immediately placed her on my abdomen and allowed the cord to finish pulsing. I remember being exhausted and crying with happiness. It was all a big blur. She was here at last—a little bloody, but beautiful and healthy. I was … tired, … [but I] had no medication whatsoever. My labor had started at two in the morning, and she arrived at five in the afternoon. It was a long day.

To have my husband involved in his child's birth, we took Bradley classes during the pregnancy, and read Leboyer's book, *Birth Without Violence*. As it turned out, Jeff wasn't able to do as much as I hoped—it just wasn't possible for him to be the kind of birth coach I envisioned. So giving our daughter her first bath was an opportunity for him to bond with our new baby in a memorable, intimate way.

The doctor and his wife, a nurse midwife, made a little ceremony of Jeff cutting the umbilical cord. They clamped off a section of the cord and graciously handed him the scissors. They said, "Now, would you like to cut your daughter free?"

He accepted, and cut the cord. Elisabeth continued to lie against my chest for a few minutes, while a nurse prepared the warm bath for her. Once the water was ninety-eight degrees, the doctor gently handed the baby to her dad. The tub for the baby was a round, plastic wash basin, placed on a counter in a corner of the room. Jeff cradled Elisabeth and gently lifted her into the bath while the doctor looked on. Jeff didn't actually bathe her. He and his daughter just spent about five minutes looking into each other's eyes, as he lovingly held her in the water. They created a special moment in time with the Leboyer bath.

Elisabeth didn't cry during any of it. She seemed very relaxed. They brought her over to me to see if she wanted to nurse, 'cause they thought that might help to deliver the placenta. I was so tired, my nipples wouldn't go erect, and Elisabeth wasn't interested in nursing at all. She just looked at my breasts, and soon fell asleep. She was too tired and I was too tired—both of us needed some rest.

We rested for awhile, and then they encouraged me to try and nurse her again. She nursed a little bit and the placenta came out.

By about six-thirty or seven o'clock, I had stabilized and so had she, and we were able to go home. We spent our first night together at home and in bed as a threesome. Part of the night she spent nursing and in my arms, and the rest of the night she spent sleeping on her dad's chest, with skin-to-skin contact. It was a very beautiful moment for us when we had her home. We never had her taken away from us, which would have happened in a hospital. None of the routine things they do to babies was done, with the exception of drops in her eyes.

The only time she cried was when they put her on the scale to weigh her—she didn't like the scale because it was cold. As soon as she was off the scale she stopped crying.

I was very pleased with the way the birth went. She was born and never had to separate from her parents, and we were able to go home right away and establish a normal routine.

Elisabeth came through the birth well. It was everything I hoped it would be, although nobody can prepare you for back labor. That feeling of passing a watermelon sideways is indescribable—there are no words. The fact that the amniotic sac was so tough that it didn't burst was part of the problem. There was so much pressure when she entered my pelvis, along with the pressure on the sac and not having it break—that was what the discomfort was from. As soon as the water broke, things really changed. If I had known that before, I would have asked him to break the membrane sooner.

What prepared me most for the birth was doing extensive reading, including Leboyer's book on birth, and also reading Bradley's book, *Husband-Coached Childbirth.* I read every book on birth I could get my hands on. I also went to prenatal exercise classes and talked to women who were further along than I was. I was able to hear about their experiences and share my own.

Later, when they had their babies, they came back to exercise class and talked to us about their births. I found that a fascinating experience—to hear what they went through in terms of labor and delivery. These were things not found in books. Now there is a book like that, and my story is a part of it.

In the prenatal exercise classes, couples were instructed about coaching and encouraged to work as a team, so they'd know what to do when labor started. I liked these classes and hoped my husband would be drawn into them as I was.

I had a suspicion I might have a big baby because I was enormous by the end of my pregnancy. I gained thirty-five pounds and I'm only five-feet-one—I felt like a tank. I was an eight-pound baby when I was born, so I thought the possibility was there for me to have a large baby.

From the sonogram, she looked like a good-sized baby. A diagnostic ultrasound was scheduled because I had gained so much weight so fast, and there was the suspicion I might be carrying twins.

As long as a woman doesn't have any health problems, I don't see anything wrong with recommending she give birth in a birth center for a first baby. If she has problems, which are a concern to her and her obstetrician, she'll want to be very careful which birth center she chooses...or she might prefer to use an ABC room in a hospital.

If she's healthy, and this is her first birth, and there's no history of complicated deliveries in her family, then she could take one of the less medical options—like home birth. It's a lot of risk for a baby, especially a first baby, to have a home birth. So many things can go wrong in a delivery that you can't foresee. I think you'd be taking your life and your baby's life in your hands, to have a baby without an experienced medical person in attendance.

There was a hospital standing by in case I had any complication. We completed all the paperwork at the back-up hospital, in case I needed to be transferred from the birth center. I liked that feeling— the insurance of having the staff of a hospital as a back-up, but not having to deal with their bureaucracy and red tape if it wasn't necessary. A lot of women go into labor thinking they're going to have a vaginal birth and end up having a C-section. I could have been one of those women, too. I wanted to make sure if there was that kind of decision that had to be made, there'd be people I could trust to help me make that decision. It was really important for me to have an OB/GYN at the birth, not only a midwife.

Some of the reasons I like the birth center are because it's a calm environment and I could have whoever I wanted in the room. Nobody made me do anything I didn't want to do. I had the doctor and his wife, plus my husband and my childbirth teacher. I considered having another friend there, but it would have been too crowded. It isn't a very large room, and they prefer only two others to attend the birth.

I knew if I was in a hospital, they would have put a fetal monitor on me, whether I liked it or not. I didn't want that unless it was absolutely necessary, and I didn't want to lie on one of those hard delivery tables. They're torture, and I hate that.

The freedom and comfort of the birth center were marvelous. I really had the best of both worlds.... I had the quality of a home environment *with* the medical expertise. It's an intermediate place between a home birth and a hospital birth.

Also, I didn't want to have any medication or anesthesia. I didn't want to miss anything, and because of that [I] was totally committed to having a baby without medication. I knew from what I read that women had healthier babies if they didn't have any medication. An epidural was an option, but I didn't think I could function with it.

I was aware birth would be painful and unlike anything I had ever experienced in my life. It was like being in the ocean and having one wave after another coming over you, and you could barely get your head above the water before the next wave hit. I was so busy just dealing with what was happening in my body, [and] as painful as it was I didn't want to miss any of it ... especially since I knew it was better for my baby for me not to have any medication.

It was more painful than I anticipated. In the course of labor, a mystical relationship developed between me and my childbirth teacher. I concentrated so much—by staying centered and watching my breathing. When the contractions came closer together, I couldn't talk, because it was too much of an effort to formulate a sentence. All I could do was be with my body and try to react to it. The childbirth teacher was able to tune in to what I needed at the time. She held me, and knew just where to massage me. She'd get behind me, put her arm around me, and whisper sweet, wonderful things in my ear as I was going through labor. These were the things that made me feel comforted. It was like a mother holding her daughter—that's what it felt like.

She'd given birth to a daughter less than a year before, so she knew what it was like. There was this odd connection—I didn't have to tell her what I needed. She knew when back labor began— where to touch me, how to hold me, and what to say. It was very, very helpful, because she was the ideal birth coach. I just wanted to be left to my own devices—to do what felt natural to do, and have someone know what was going on to guide me, which is what she did.

She offered suggestions, like positional changes that might help; massaged my perinium with warm vitamin E oil, and did all the things that made me feel cared for and comforted. I didn't have to think about anything—she thought of almost everything for me. I didn't have to worry about having to speak to people—she just knew automatically what I wanted and needed. That's what every woman dreams of when they're giving birth to a baby. You don't have the energy to talk, at least I didn't. I was in a very meditative state, and tried to stay there. I felt that was the healthiest place to be.

My husband would come over at times and hold my hand, to participate in the birth. Even though he wasn't sure how to help me, he was supportive. Giving Elisabeth the bath, after he cut the umbilical cord, helped Jeff feel he was an integral part of the birth, and I'm glad he had that experience.

One piece of advice I'd give women before they get pregnant, is to get in really good physical condition. I thought I was, but it turned out I wasn't. The labor took much more out of me than I expected it would. If I had been in better physical condition and more toned, I'm sure I wouldn't have been so tired. If I had it to do over again, I would gain much less weight and exercise all the way through the pregnancy. You feel more like exercising when you're not so heavy. Since you don't know how long your labor's going to go, expect a marathon and pray for a sprint.

Also, watch your nutritional intake. I followed Adele Davis's, *Let's Have Healthy Babies,* and I gained a lot of weight because I ate liver almost every day, and lots of dairy products. I had rich, raw milk, and all these cheeses and yogurts. You might want to be careful about your diet, because putting on all those extra pounds made it more difficult for me to exercise and keep in shape while I was pregnant. I felt like the Goodyear Blimp, and I looked like it, too. So it's a good idea not to gain too much weight.

The vitamin E oil was a good trick—be sure to massage it into the tissues so the skin will become more elastic. It's great to avoid having an episiotomy that way. And Leboyer had a lovely idea for having a more humane, sensitive birth—low lights, quiet voices, and a warm bath for the newborn. We're glad we did it that way.

138

Introduction to Chapter 15

Water Birth in a Birth Center

In the following story, a couple plans a birth center birth for their first baby. They also know there's a possibility for them to have the baby born underwater—a water birth. The woman labors part of the time in water, usually the last hour or more, and delivers underwater.

There are two types of water birth: "rapid-emergence water births" where as soon as the entire baby is in the water, he or she is lifted out and placed on the mother's chest or abdomen; and "slow-emergence water births" in which the baby is allowed to stay underwater for several minutes, until the cord stops pulsing. In both cases, the placenta should be delivered out of the water, to see that it's all in one piece.

The rapid-emergence water birth is the type being discussed in the following story. This kind of water birth is more commonly practiced, because there is less risk of the placenta separating while the mother is in the water. The longer the cord-cutting is delayed, the less oxygen there is for the baby because blood can pool between the uterine wall and the buckled placenta once the baby is born, cutting its oxygen supply.

The reason it is suggested that women using the birth center not enter the tub too early in labor (before five to seven centimeters), is that the water can have a narcotic effect and slow down labor. There are, however, some women who can enter the tub at five centimeters and deliver an hour later. Women generally relax in the water, allowing the cervix to open, often quite rapidly. Many push for only a half-hour, and then deliver their babies.

Some women find water birth to have the following advantages: reduces pain during the latter stage of labor; accelerates cervical dilation upon entering the water, especially when the woman is already at seven centimeters; freedom of movement; encourages the woman to have more control over her birth; a sharp decrease in anesthetics, Pitocin, forceps, and unnecessary C-sections.

Technical Reference: *Pre- & Peri-Natal Psychology News, Volume II, Issue I, Spring, 1988, Steven Raymond, R.N., Editor*

Donna

Donna and her husband planned to have their first baby in a free-standing birth center, unaffiliated with a hospital. The baby was born underwater after three days of labor, and was delivered by Donna and her husband.

As a nurse, I saw a lot of babies born when I went through nurse's training. Most of them were forceps deliveries, and they were all women who had medication during labor. Some of them had spinals, and some of them had epidurals. In either case, they couldn't feel when they were pushing.

I saw my sister-in-law's baby born in the birth center where we chose to have our first baby. I took pictures for her at the birth. I thought it was a wonderful experience, in comparison to what I saw as a student nurse. I became interested in having a baby, pretty soon after my husband and I were married. As time went on, we became more serious about it.

I liked the "non-intervention" approach of the birth center, letting the woman do everything by herself. She didn't have to be on a table, in stirrups, heavily medicated, with the doctor yanking the baby out, which is literally what I saw in hospitals where I worked.

Our daughter was born September 24, and was our first baby. I came to the birth center three times a week for prenatal exercise classes. When women had their babies, they'd drop out for awhile, and then come back and talk about their birth experiences. They'd bring their babies in when they returned, and continue coming to classes to get back in shape after birth.

When I heard different women talking about labor and delivery, I was sure I'd be able to have a baby without medication. Since I was able to film Mary's birth, I saw what it could be like under the best circumstances. She didn't have her baby born in water, but she was squatting when she delivered. She always seemed to stay in control during labor. Actually, she became so relaxed between contractions, she fell asleep. You could see her body's endorphin system was working perfectly.

I think that's what made me feel comfortable about a non-medicated birth. I heard from many women who achieved natural childbirth, and they loved it. I had seen it for myself and wasn't worried when it was time for me to give birth.

When I was three weeks overdue, and didn't have any signs of labor, I thought I'd have to go to the hospital, and I was *so set* on having the birth in the birthing center.

In case I had to be transferred to a hospital from the birth center, I was required to take classes at the hospital across the street to prepare for using their alternative birthing center (ABC) room. My insurance didn't cover the birth center, so I was really torn between whether ... to have the baby at the center, or in the hospital's birthing unit.

To decide, I went to the classes and on a tour of the hospital. The birthing unit is always busy, because there's only one birthing room, so the chances of being able to give birth there are slim. In fact, every time I'd go there, it was being used and I couldn't see it.

When I saw all the machines used on the obstetrical floor of the hospital, I knew what my decision would be—with all those monitors and technical electronics, I'd be less scared in the birth center. I was really frightened ... as I was more and more overdue. [I was afraid] that I'd end up having the baby in the hospital, and my labor would be induced.

According to my calculations, she was three weeks overdue, but after five non-stress tests and five diagnostic ultrasounds, they determined she was only a day or two overdue. My due date was evidently off. I didn't have an ultrasound until the last three weeks of my pregnancy because I was healthy, and I was pretty sure about the date of conception.

The doctor broke the amniotic sac when I came into the birth center. I had already been in false labor, on and off, for three days. He said I had been in labor long enough, and he broke my water to help speed things up. It took me about five hours to go from four centimeters to seven centimeters.

In the beginning of labor I had a lot of back pain, but I normally have back problems, so it wasn't back labor. I also had low contractions around my stomach. When I had a contraction, my

141

husband put a heating pad on my back. I couldn't lie down at all. I had one contraction lying down after the nurse checked me, and I couldn't get up fast enough—it was more painful in that position.

For most of the contractions after that, and because I'm so tall, I put one of the center's little step stools on a counter, and then a pillow on top of that. I labored leaning forward over the counter. I'd just breathe through my contractions. I learned different kinds of breathing from the classes, but I think I used my own method. My body adjusted to the pain level—breathed faster when I was in more pain. That's basically how I got through labor.

When I was dilated seven centimeters, I went into the tub. As soon as I sat down, my back pain was gone. Once I was in the tub, it took me only an hour to get to ten centimeters. When I had my first contraction in the tub, it was still very painful. My husband was taking washcloths and squeezing water over my back. The feeling of the water dripping on my back was so relaxing. The water was only up to my waist, so I liked the added feeling of the water down my back.

My husband was just terrific! He played an active role in the birth, and that was a high point. The nurse who assisted us knew my husband—they went to high school together. It was like a big family affair, and we were very comfortable with her there. She didn't do much except check the baby's heartbeat and my cervical dilation.

When I was ready to push, I held onto the bars they have on the sides of the tub while I squatted. My husband was sitting in the tub behind me. Between contractions, I would lean against his knees. At one point, I had a contraction and I could feel the baby's head coming. I reached down and I could feel her head, although she wasn't out yet.

My husband's sister went to get the doctor. He came in, and asked if I saw the head or had just felt it.

And I said, "Well, I felt it."

The doctor said, "Oh well, you just felt it. You know it's usually a long time from crowning until the head's delivered."

So the next contraction, he was looking with a flashlight in the water, and said, "No, I don't see anything. Oh my gosh, there's the whole head."

142

Her head came out in one contraction. After that it was really neat.... My husband reached down and felt her ear and her hair—which was very soft in the water. I felt her head.

And then, during the next contraction, as I pushed my husband kept his hands under the water. He gently guided her, when her body was out, and pushed her up. Then I reached down and grabbed her out of the water. So the doctor never touched her.

She was never taken away from me after she was born. The doctor suctioned out her nose and mouth. She was a little blue, but she cried right away and she was fine. I stayed in the tub for about twenty minutes after she was born. Then my husband cut the cord and I got out. I started having contractions because I hadn't delivered the placenta, and they want you to be out of the tub when that happens so they can check that it's all in one piece.

It was fantastic for us to deliver our own baby! When I first heard about this birthing center, I was a little leery about it, especially since I came from a medical background. I was concerned about problems that might happen during labor or delivery.

Many friends told us to wait until we had a second baby to deliver there. They said, "After you have one baby, and you know everything went fine, then you can go to a birthing center. You shouldn't have your first one there."

After my sister-in-law had her first baby at the center, I saw it was possible for me to do the same thing. If I became a high-risk patient during the course of my pregnancy, then I'd be carefully watched to determine if I could still deliver at the center or have to go across the street to the hospital.

In order to give birth at the birthing center, a woman has to have a healthy pregnancy and no signs of diabetes or high blood pressure. And the doctor doesn't normally make deliveries in the birth center when a woman is more than two weeks post-term. I was so frightened about going to the hospital, and had my mind set on delivering in the birth center. I joked with my doctor that if I couldn't use the birth center, I was going to deliver at home and call him when it was over—I was that determined to be at the center.

The Monday before I gave birth, the doctor did a hysteroscopy. He went up through the cervix with a scope and looked at the amniotic fluid in the sac, to make sure there wasn't any meconium, and that it wasn't green, which meant the baby was in distress. The fluid was clear and looked fine, so he let me continue with the pregnancy.

I liked that we were allowed to have our birth the way we wanted. If I wanted to walk around, I walked around. If I wanted to lie down, I laid down, although not too many women do that.

When I talked to women who had their babies in the hospital, they said, "I don't think I could have walked."

I don't think I could have laid in bed like they did. I think it's because they're told not to walk that they believe they couldn't.

When I had a contraction, I'd be thinking, "Thank you for not slowing down," especially when I got in the water. There are times when women get in the water and their contractions slow down. Then they have to get out of the tub. That's the reason you have to wait until your cervix has dilated seven centimeters.

When I first went in the tub, the doctor said, "If you get in the water now, you're going to have to get out again before you deliver, and then get back in. Otherwise, you'll be a prune by the time you deliver."

I said, "I don't care, I want to get in the water."

The baby was born within an hour after that, perhaps because I relaxed so much. For my next baby, I'd like to labor at home in the bathtub...because it was so comfortable.

I didn't experience the so called "transition" phase of labor—when the contractions keep building, one on top of the other, like waves following each other to the shore. Many women experience this, feeling like they'll never be able to catch up. I never felt that way, because I went into the water just before "transition" and ... [the water] relaxed me so much. The contractions were coming faster, but they didn't feel a lot stronger. I kept thinking, "Oh good, I'm having another contraction—I can stay in the water."

We had the birth videotaped so we can look back on it. I didn't want to do that at first, but I'm really glad we did—we've watched it many times. I've shown it to friends, although some women friends think I'm crazy, because I gave birth in water [at a birth center] instead of in a hospital. And then, when they hear my husband and I delivered the baby ourselves, they can't believe it. One of the nurses I work with now, who handles high-risk mothers and babies, saw the videotape. She was in awe, watching me give birth—it was so different from the way she sees women give birth in hospitals.

Attending the exercise classes helped me prepare for childbirth. I went three times a week, and started when I was about two months pregnant. I saw the actual birthing rooms in early pregnancy, when I came to the classes, since they were held in the birth center. Seeing the rooms where I'd give birth was exciting, and motivated me to have a healthy pregnancy so I could ... [go] there.

Exercising all through pregnancy, and being supervised by an instructor who is trained in prenatal exercise, is very important, and it helps build stamina. You should never get your heart rate over a hundred and forty when you're pregnant. After your first trimester, you're not supposed to do exercises lying on your back, because your uterus is too heavy on your aorta. It cuts down the blood supply to yourself and to the baby. Aerobic exercises should be modified to low-impact aerobics. Swimming and walking are both fine when you're pregnant.

When I thought I was overdue, I walked five to six times a day, trying to get that baby to come out. Now I know babies come out when they're ready—you can't force them out by walking.

I think taking exercise classes helped increase my stamina. Over the three days I was in labor, I got very little sleep. I probably slept four hours the whole time. The first night, I didn't sleep at all. The second night, I may have slept four hours. I went home after I saw the doctor on Tuesday and tried to go to sleep, but the phone kept ringing and different things distracted me from sleeping.

I knew I was going to be back at the birthing center the next day. I was worried about that, because I guess I thought the doctor might tell me to go to the hospital. When I started having contractions and they weren't *that* close together, I wanted my husband to time them, but he thought they were too far apart.

The exercise classes helped me with pushing, since we did a lot of abdominal exercises. I actually used too much force, and tore myself a little. That was because her head came out so quickly, and I couldn't control the pushing once I felt the urge to push. I remember pushing and moaning and saying, "Oh, it hurts, it hurts."

And the nurse told me to stop pushing, but I couldn't stop myself because my body took over. I probably should have done some breathing then, if I really didn't want to tear. Pushing was all I could think of at the moment, and my husband wanted to help me get her out. He didn't even think about saying, "Do some different breathing and try not to push."

I watched a Lamaze video just before I had our baby. My husband rented it, 'cause he thought we should practice the breathing, and it might make me more comfortable. It was the worst thing in the world. The woman ended up giving birth flat on her back, with an IV, and had an episiotomy. That film depicted a typical birth for a woman in a large hospital in most cities in the United States. I knew I didn't want to have a birth like that.

One piece of advice, which might help women, is "plan for the baby to be late." I know two other women whose babies were due right around the time mine was. They both gave birth before me. When I didn't go into labor when I expected to, it was very hard on me. I kept wanting it to start. I never thought this baby would be late. Women should count on their babies being two weeks late, and really set that in their minds. The waiting is the hardest thing. I felt like a time bomb. I'd think, "When is this going to happen? Is it safe to go to the grocery store. Is my water going to break?"

I didn't gain much, only fifteen pounds. The small amount of weight also helped me feel healthy. I ate very well and stayed away from junk food and empty calories. I didn't smoke or drink at any time during the pregnancy. For peace of mind, I think women should not drink any alcohol when they're pregnant. If there's a birth defect, you won't blame yourself. But if you had a baby diagnosed with fetal alcohol syndrome, who else could you blame if you'd been drinking?

I think it's important for women to have the birth they want. If you want to give birth in a birthing center, and perhaps have an underwater birth, then that's fine. If you want to have the baby in a hospital, with an IV ... [and a] choice of medications, and possibly use stirrups for delivery, I think it's fine for people who want to have it that way.

The most important thing is for women to be comfortable in their minds and in their bodies. If ... [the mother's] frightened, or feeling uneasy about the lack of equipment and monitors in the birthing center, then she should be in a hospital where ... [everything is available for] intervention if ... [she needs] it.

I didn't have any fear about labor at the birthing center. I felt so comfortable, because I was there three times a week for the exercise classes. It became a second home to me. My sister-in-law was active in the birthing center, helping out the staff with different things. I was able to come in at any time. I brought my mother in to show her around. She wasn't crazy about me giving birth there, but she accepted my decision. She said, "I would never do it that way, but if that's what you want, then that's fine."

When we decided to film the birth, we set the camcorder on a tripod in the corner of the birthing room we used, and it did it's own thing—we didn't have to worry about it. My sister-in-law took some snapshots during labor and delivery.

I also had a friend at the birth, who had given birth at the center a month earlier—it was her second child. She was the most helpful to me. She came to our house when I was in the beginning of labor. At first, I was uncomfortable with her being there, 'cause it was like another presence and our house is very small. As time went on, she knew just where to rub my back, and what to say to me, and she stayed four hours.

When I returned to the birth center for the second time, on the third day of labor, I called her and asked if she'd join us. She knew what I was going through.... [She was] a tremendous help because she had been through two births herself, both at the birthing center, and her most recent was in the water, too.

Vaginal Birth After Cesarean (VBAC)

A woman who had a cesarean section, and wants to attempt a vaginal birth, such as the woman in the following story, is not as rare as it was ten years ago. There are few reasons why a woman shouldn't attempt a vaginal birth after a cesarean, and the most important risk is the type of incision that was made on the uterus. If it was a classical (vertical) incision there's a slightly higher chance of uterine rupture (bursting of the uterus) during labor, than if it was a horizontal cut. However, the incidence of uterine rupture during a vaginal attempt is less than four percent, which is extremely low.

Beginning in the eighties, mothers who had previously had C-sections, and were about to have second babies, sometimes tried for VBACs, generally with a doctor who had a high (at least eighty percent) success rate.

Some doctors require an IV be hooked up, as a condition of attempting a VBAC in a hospital, in case medications become necessary during labor or delivery.

A woman was labeled "high risk" if she had had a previous cesarean, and usually was not allowed to attempt a VBAC in a birth center. Some women are successful with VBACs at home, but most doctors would consider that extremely risky and dangerous. Times are changing, though, and many less repeat cesareans are scheduled than were ten years ago.

The phrase, "Once a cesarean, always a cesarean," was popularized by Dr. Cragin in 1916, in hopes that doctors would refrain from performing unnecessary C-sections, since he believed once one was done the following births had to be surgical deliveries. Since 1980, more than eighty percent of the attempted vaginal births, after one or more cesareans, have been achieved. Dr. Cragin's statement is ancient history.

Technical Reference: *Laurence D. Colman, M.D., specializing in Obstetrics, Gynecology, Infertility, and Endocrinology, Santa Monica, California*

Lauren

Lauren was thirty-three-years-old when she gave birth to her second child, vaginally, after having her first child by cesarean section two years earlier.

For my first baby, I planned a normal delivery in the birth center. I wanted to have its homey atmosphere. Before that pregnancy, I looked for a doctor who wasn't quick to do a C-section. The doctor we chose held out as long as I was willing to, which really helped—I didn't have to argue with my doctor in addition to everything else going on.

When my contractions began, we went to the birth center and the staff was very supportive. When they … [assisted] me, it was like they were saying, "Try a little longer." My labor went on for hours and hours. I walked; got on all fours; sat up on the bed; kept changing positions to try to get comfortable. The baby was posterior and wouldn't turn over. After about a day and a half, I didn't care if it hurt more, I just wanted to lie down. I was so tired.

Then the doctor said it would probably be another day before I got to ten centimeters—if I ever would.

I said, "I can't go on another day."

So they wrote on my chart, "Reason for Transfer: Failure to Progress." The word "failure" really bothered me. Why is it always our fault? The labels are a real drawback. I wish they'd come up with some other way of phrasing it.

The care was totally different in the hospital. They put the monitor on me and ordered me to, "Lift your hips." They seemed oblivious to the fact that I was in the middle of a contraction.

I said, "Please, you'll have to wait until the contraction is over."

They started pulling the monitor strap that was around my belly, trying to get it out from under me. I had no trouble cooperating, I just wanted them to wait until I was through with the

150

contraction. I said, *"You* wait!" I got really angry and they backed off.

They acted in the same manner when they transferred me into the operating room, rushing me onto the gurney while I was having a contraction, and I told them they had to wait until it was over.

It was the first time I'd ever been in a hospital, so I don't know whether their behavior was typical or not. It certainly wasn't very personal, and I didn't know they had to come and harass you every hour or so for your temperature and vital signs.

The actual experience in the operating room was no big deal. After an hour, the nightmare was over. Their attitude was what upset me. They didn't explain what they were doing or what was happening to me.

After the C-section, my husband went to the nursery with the baby, and they put me in "recovery." He told me I was there about an hour and a-half, all by myself. In that whole time, one person came to check on me. Otherwise, I just laid there, kind of in a fog.

When I was taken to my room, he came in and said he'd been in the nursery holding Katherine and rocking her. I felt very deprived. Later I had a different perspective on it because I knew I'd be with her the rest of our lives, and I'd have other kids. But that's a special time, when they're first born. I got to enjoy that the second time—with my son.

The first couple [of] days after my daughter's birth, I didn't feel like a mother. It seemed to have happened to someone else, not me. I think that's why it took so long to reconcile [myself to] the C-section.... With my son, the next day I was a little dazed, but it was like I was watching myself— not someone else.

Before the first baby, the classes we took prepared us only for a normal birth. They covered the procedures for a C-section, but they didn't talk about how you'd feel—you know, that you might feel disappointed.

It may have been just the change from before I had a baby— being able to do whatever I wanted, when I wanted—to being responsible for someone. I was depressed for about six weeks. That was a long time, and the only way I knew to treat it was by thinking to myself, "I'll get through this day." I would have been more active if I hadn't had a cesarean. Activity helps fight depression. Eventually it lifted, but it was hard.

My husband kept saying, "Think about the pregnancy. You didn't have any water retention; you were really healthy; you've got a great baby now. Why are you unhappy?"

He just couldn't understand, and I eventually got to the point where I didn't even try to talk to him. That made it worse 'cause then I buried my feelings. It took four or five months for me to accept the reality of what had happened.

I knew that support groups were in existence, and I knew there were places to go where I could talk about it, but I felt I could deal with it, and eventually I did. I'm sure it took longer than it would have if I'd gone and talked with people who understood, who'd been through what I'd been through.

I think you can have high expectations, but if I had it to do over again, I'd pay attention to the class discussion of C-sections, instead of dismissing the possibility that it could happen to me. After all, I buckle my seatbelt every time I get in the car. I've never been in an accident, but I still buckle it.

My advice to women having their first babies would be to *prepare for the possibility of having a C-section.* We went over it in class and then I tuned it out, like it's not going to be me. And then it was me. I was so unprepared.

They told us the procedures and what would happen, but they didn't really talk about how we'd feel emotionally. They didn't talk about emotions at all. The teacher was ecstatic about babies, and made us think they'd just hand us our baby, and then sew me up. Instead, it took a couple of weeks after the birth before I was thrilled about having a baby.

For expectant couples, I'd say, "Check out the hospital and the rules, and everything governing C-sections and visitation, etc." We took a tour of part of the hospital and saw the alternative birth center room. We weren't sure we wanted to be there or at the birth center. As it turned out, we weren't in either, and I had totally dismissed the idea of being in a hospital.

We should have prepared for the hospital experience by taking a complete tour of the maternity facilities, because we didn't even know where the nursery was.

Second Birth: VBAC

I knew, after having the first baby, I'd try for a vaginal birth with my second. It just didn't occur to me not to. I figured, "OK, it wasn't for the first, but we'll try it with the next."

I got a lot of support from our doctor, however my husband didn't encourage me to have a VBAC (vaginal birth after cesarean). He felt I'd placed too much emphasis on our daughter being a cesarean instead of a vaginal baby. I understood he couldn't relate to my feelings, so I didn't even try to discuss it with him. I thought that was the best approach, because I knew the doctors and nurses were on my side.

Everyone in our family wanted to know whether I was going to have another cesarean. You know, "Once a cesarean, always a cesarean."

We answered, "No, we're going to try the other way."

They'd say, "Oh, okay," and drop it. That made it easy. They didn't say, "You can't do that."

While I was pregnant with my second child, I was pretty active chasing after our daughter. We didn't attend the childbirth classes. It wasn't a requirement since we had gone to the first ones. We rarely did any breathing exercises or anything like that. If I got my husband to do them with me once a week, it was a lot. I thought, "Well, this time, why fight it?" So I didn't.

Very late, he got into the spirit of having our second baby. When the baby was a week overdue, he called me on the phone and said, "Do you think tonight we should do some of those exercises?" I just laughed.

Just about everything was different for the second birth. My son's head was down, facing my back, so the labor pain was all in front. With the first birth—my daughter—the entire labor was in my lower back, because her head pressed against my spine.

This time, as the contractions got stronger, I convinced myself it wasn't going to work. They had given me a shot of Stadol at the birth center, to let me get some rest, so we went home and I fell asleep. I woke up with each contraction, and as soon as it was over, went to sleep again. There wasn't any relaxing and recovering. All of a sudden, I'd wake up in the middle of a contraction without any preparation time.

After an hour of that, the shot wore off. I was having trouble dealing with the contractions, because they were coming one right on top of the other. At that point, my husband decided that we better have a C-section. He called the center and said, "She can't stand the contractions anymore. We're going to the hospital and get this over with."

Both of us were thinking about the last time when I was in labor thirty hours, so this time it'll take thirty hours and we can't go that long with this type of labor. However, at the thought of a cesarean, I just went to pieces. They could hear me over the phone—"No, I don't want a C-section, I want to go on."

When I was in labor with our first baby, I had more support from my husband. I think we were more naive and expected it would take only about eight hours to give birth. There were also differences in what I needed from my husband during labor. For the first one, at the birth center, my husband put his hands on either side of my spine, putting pressure on it, and that helped to relieve the pain.

With the second one, there was nothing for him to do. At home, he asked between contractions, "Is there anything I can do to make this easier?"

I was in such pain, all I could do was scream, "No, don't touch me." I think I tried just about every position. I tried standing, leaning against the wall, on my knees, leaning against the bed. The only thing I didn't try was getting on all fours. There wasn't a single position that lessened the pain or made it more comfortable, but being able to try them all helped.

Then we went to the birth center, and when they examined me, I was eight centimeters dilated. A couple hours earlier, I had been only two centimeters dilated. When they said I was eight centimeters, I couldn't believe it.

I sat there and the water broke. Everyone got excited and said, "Look at her, she's smiling." It was no problem from then on 'cause I knew I could do it. I was over the hump.

During labor, just before transition my husband was sitting on the bed with me leaning between his legs, I remember asking, "Is this going to work?" I really felt anytime they would say, "No, it won't work. Let's go to the hospital." I could hear the chuckles, too, so I thought my question must not have sounded too brilliant.

Everyone said, "Yes, it will work."

I think what really helped toward the end was, when we were trying different positions, the doctor said, "Well, why don't you sit on the toilet?... That puts you in a natural position for birth."

We did, and in just one or two contractions, my baby's head came out, then the body, and it felt good. It was much easier using that squat method. I think I was actually on the toilet while I was pushing the head out. The doctor said I had to stand up to push out the body. I must have had some support 'cause I know I was fairly upright, with my knees bent. I think my husband was holding me up from behind, while the doctor caught the baby.

With him, labor lasted about fourteen hours—half the time of my first. Right after our son was born, my husband cut the cord and my baby was wrapped in a towel and handed to me while I was still sitting on the toilet. After a while, the nurse took him to clean him up while I made my way to the bed. When he was clean, they brought him to me [again]. It was a wonderful feeling to have him there while we both rested and just looked at one another. This time, I was with my baby immediately after the birth— instead of being separated from him.... The bond between us was firmly formed instantly.

Our son's birth validated both experiences. It's strange, but his seemed to make up for hers. Like having one baby vaginally made up for having the other one cesarean. I could go on from there.

I was home seven or eight hours after he was born. I told people that, and they thought I was crazy to come home so quickly. When I was in the hospital with my daughter, I didn't get any rest. They were constantly checking on me after surgery, every hour or two.

Our son woke us up just once the first night. He nursed and went back to sleep, so we got almost a full night's rest, and I was able to be with our two-year-old daughter.

I'm doing much better after the second birth. In fact, my husband stayed home the first week, and my mother-in-law came for the next week. She kept telling me to stay in bed and rest. I thought, "I can't stay in bed another day!" I felt so good, I wanted to be up doing things.

With perspective on the two births, I can compare how my husband and I handled the two labors. When I was in labor with our first child, my husband wanted to be the coach. I wouldn't let him, because we hadn't practiced any exercises beforehand. He never learned the accelerated breathing pattern. We weren't a team, but he tried to make us one, and I resented that.

For the second birth, we didn't even try to do the exercises, but his presence and encouraging words helped me along and we did a lot better. So I'd say if you haven't practiced being a team, don't change it in the middle of labor. That really threw me off. It's important to work together and plan ... or just be there and hold her hand.

I know my husband was concerned that I might have another cesarean. Recently, we talked about how he felt—something we didn't do after our daughter was born.

We went through so much during the first labor. With the second one, by the time the contractions were unmanageable, my husband wanted to have the C-section—get it over with. Because the first one turned out okay, for him anyway, he didn't want to deal with having to keep trying for a vaginal birth. That's where we differed. In the middle of labor is no time to talk about that.

I really hadn't thought about what birth would be like before I had the first baby. I think my mother was very inhibited. She didn't even inform me about menstruation. Thank God for the classes in school. However ill-prepared those are, they're better than nothing.

Maybe Mom did me some favors and disfavors by not telling me about childbirth, 'cause I didn't have any preconceptions. So when I went into it, the VBAC anyway, I knew what it was supposed to be, but had no idea how it would feel. All I knew was that having a vaginal birth was very important to me.

Part IV
HOME BIRTH

Introduction to Chapter 17

First Baby Born at Home

Many women feel they'll be more content giving birth at home than in a hospital or birth center. In the following story, a home birth was chosen because it seemed a natural place with more comfort and control.

Deciding to be at home requires the couple to take more responsibility than they would have in a hospital or birth center. That's because they won't be able to use any medications at home, and will have to decide how to handle a drug-free labor and delivery. Please see the "Introduction to Chapter 18," for a detailed list of deterrents to home birth. Those risks require the availability of medical back-up. Knowing the distance from home to emergency medical help, and other specific back-up plans need to be made, in the event they are required.

The advantages of home birth include: reduced costs for labor, delivery, and postpartum; more choices during labor, in terms of mobility, eating, and drinking; any number of people you want at the birth; more self-control over the delivery; no interference by medical personnel or procedures; not having the baby taken away from you after birth; less risk of infection than in the hospital; less anxiety for women who are fearful of hospitals and their procedures; having other children at the birth.

Deciding to give birth at home means using a midwife rather than a doctor, because medical insurance companies refuse to insure a family practitioner who does home births, and some will refuse to insure a doctor who works with a midwife. Midwives are more familiar with home births than doctors. Most doctors have never seen a birth without some medical intervention, whereas midwives are more familiar with a non-intervention approach to birth.

It's important for couples planning a home birth to attend a childbirth preparation class. The most popular courses are Lamaze and Bradley. The main difference between them is that one has an external focus (Lamaze), and the other an internal focus (Bradley), during labor.

The Lamaze method teaches couples how to use specific breathing techniques, as a way to distract the laboring woman from the painful contractions. These are diaphragm-breathing methods which combine exhaling and inhaling at different intervals, for the various stages of labor. Lamaze also suggests the woman keep her eyes on a photograph or drawing (a "focal point") on a nearby wall, to absorb her concentration when each contraction begins. And a form of massaging the abdomen, called "effleurage," is used to calm the laboring woman, especially during early labor. Another part of Lamaze training is learning how to relax one part of the body when another part is rigid, to simulate what happens during the contractions of the uterus. Her support person, or "coach," will simulate a contraction by squeezing a part of her body while she relaxes a particular part, such as her right arm or right leg, following the applied pressure. With practice, she learns how to relax any part of her body when the squeeze technique is used.

In the Bradley method, women use only abdominal breathing, and they discover ways to relax their bodies and minds while contractions are being timed by the instructor or coach. Rather than learning different breathing techniques or looking outside of themselves to cope with labor, women learn to use visualization, self-hypnosis or meditation as a way to diminish pain. Bradley is a more individualized method of childbirth preparation, and works well for people who need or want a less-structured approach.

To best find out about these methods, read about them or listen to personal accounts of others' experiences using the courses. It may also be possible to attend one of the classes, or to call the instructor to get questions answered and learn more about her qualifications as a childbirth educator.

(Please see the Bibliography for suggested books.)

Technical Reference: *Laurence D. Colman, M.D., specializing in Obstetrics, Gynecology, Infertility, and Endocrinology, Santa Monica, California*

Barbara

Barbara was twenty-seven when she and her husband planned to have their first baby at home, using midwives from a local birth center.

We had been married only two months when I found out I was pregnant. The first thing we had to decide was whether we wanted to keep this baby. Once we decided we wanted to, we had to choose where we wanted to give birth.

A good friend of mine, who's also from England, was pregnant at the same time, two weeks ahead of me. She planned on having her baby born at home, using midwives through a local birth center. The more I thought about it, the more it made sense—I had been born at home, and a lot of women from my mother's generation … [in England] … had home births with midwives assisting them.

Of my birth, my mother says, "It was a very cozy affair, with a lovely Irish midwife. Your dad cooked breakfast, and he had a cup of tea for me when it was all over. There was a warm feeling about it."

She said I was a sweet, calm baby, whereas my sister, who was born in a hospital some years before me, had been a difficult baby. My parents believed the birth environments influenced our personalities, but I don't believe that now, since I've given birth.

Hospitals frightened me. I'd never been in one, and my image was of steel and glass, needles and knives—things that hurt. That, to me, was a lot more frightening than giving birth at home. In fact, I never thought about that as a scary thing, although later a lot of women told me it is to them.

When I went to the birth center for our pregnancy test, I fell in love with the place immediately. It's a very reassuring atmosphere, but my husband encouraged me to have our baby at home. And since my mother did it, I thought I could too.

161

One of the first things I discussed with the midwife was my fear of having an episiotomy. The midwife said, "Oh, don't worry about that. It's a long way off."

The birth was a traumatic event, as I suppose all births are. I read throughout my pregnancy, and I was so curious to find out what birth would be like. I think the curiosity took me through a lot of it. It didn't really matter how much it hurt—I wanted to know what it felt like.

It was very painful; I won't say it wasn't. The women at the birth center didn't talk about the pain. They understated it, which I think was quite helpful.

I felt confident and excited about the event. I felt like I could do it. As the due date approached, I didn't feel quite of this world anymore. I felt elevated and distant from everybody and I didn't know what it was going to be like. I wasn't really scared, however I felt it would take courage.

The beginning of labor is fuzzy in my memory. Since she was twelve days past the due date, I took some castor oil to bring on labor. My midwife said it was okay to do that. I had about twelve to eighteen hours of mild contractions, so I couldn't sleep.

During that beginning phase, I didn't know I was in labor. I experienced a lot of discomfort and pain. It was a negative kind of feeling because I didn't know *that* was labor. The sensation of contractions were, to me, like really bad nausea, like when you're sick and feel like throwing up. I felt locked in it, knowing it was going to happen again and again.

Then the midwife came, and the contractions stopped as soon as she walked through the door. She made me feel like a sham. I got upset with the whole thing. She advised me to drink a little whiskey and go to sleep.

When I woke up after a couple of hours, the contractions started again, but this time they were very different. This time they really hurt. I no longer knew whether I was in labor or not. Because it hadn't started suddenly, I didn't know anymore. Also, my water hadn't broken. I think I was waiting for that to happen as an official sign that labor had begun. I bled with every contraction, but that didn't worry me.

Laboring for a good twelve hours without the midwife was not very pleasant, especially not knowing I was in labor. Once I was examined, and told that everything was moving along, I felt quite happy, in fact rather jolly, between contractions. I even cracked a few jokes, but they were kind of nervous jokes.

The midwife's assistant arrived first, and gave me a piece of helpful advice. She asked me to try and imagine the pelvic muscles between the contractions, and not to tighten them up, but to keep them open. That imagery helped a lot. She held my hand through each contraction, and my husband held my other hand. That's what I needed—personal contact. You have to do it by yourself, but it's so nice to hang onto somebody when you're going through it.

I sat up throughout labor. I wasn't comfortable on the bed, lying down. I couldn't understand how anyone could be comfortable lying down. I wasn't comfortable lying down through my pregnancy. It struck me as silly to be in that position. I did a bit of walking but I was happiest sitting, and I even sat on the toilet toward the end of labor. I needed a seat with a hole because, at the end, it was like sitting on a ball.

My only regret was we hadn't arranged for someone to take photographs. Other than that, I think it was very nice the way it was. We didn't have any music or set a stage with candles. I didn't feel I needed a stage to perform on; that probably would have embarrassed me. You know how it is when you go into somebody else's house, even just to visit. You lose some power—you're in someone's sphere. You're much stronger on your own ground. Imagine going to this horrible, frightening place to give birth. You lose all your power. *That's* what you need to give birth. It's a very forceful, intense experience and you need your own personal power.

I would like to have known more about the impact of children on marriage. It just amazes me how little we know about becoming parents. I don't think anyone's really prepared, and maybe no one can be until he or she becomes one. The first three months were the hardest for us, but the whole first year was quite difficult. Amy was an active baby and cried a lot.

I'm still amazed we made it. The whole birth thing astonishes me. I would like to do it again just to re-witness what I went through. Just to go back there and see it again. Maybe a second time I'd be a little more in control. All that time—the first twelve hours when I felt I'd be in agony forever—I could have eliminated that for a start. That was a question I used to ask women who had babies, "Did you know when you were in labor?" It's funny to me that I asked that question repeatedly, because as it turned out I really didn't know when my labor started.

I think I chose exactly the right method and did the best I could. I would do it again the same way. My English friend, who had her baby three weeks before I did, had a fast labor. We compared notes and we had very different pregnancies and births. I assumed I would have a longer labor, and I did. Both my mother and my sister had rather long labors, so I assumed mine would be too.

It was a humbling experience. I didn't know how to give birth and, surprisingly, it happened smoothly. There I was with a brand-new human being, somewhat in our own image. It was a very spiritual experience, even a religious experience; although I'm not a religious person.

The last twenty minutes were very difficult—I was in a lot of pain, and I started to get more vocal. This was unusual because throughout labor I had been pretty quiet. This had been an issue of mine because I was afraid of getting loud and out of control.

I didn't have the urge to push when the midwife told me I was fully dilated. But at the beginning of the next contraction, she encouraged us to start. We pushed, pushed, pushed, and I felt good about that. I was pushing harder and harder each time. I knew I was getting to the point where I was really getting into it. There was a part of me that was a bit shocked by the force of it. I felt like an animal, and it began to hurt a lot.

Then the crowning of her head caused tremendous pain. That was a fear of mine even when I was a young girl. I can remember thinking, "Imagine a great big baby coming through that little hole!" When it was actually happening, I was aware "this is the moment—this is what it's all about, and this is the bit that's really going to hurt." And it did!

Between contractions, when her head was crowning and I had to wait for the next one, I felt I was in a horrible position. I was sitting in my husband's lap and I just wanted to run away from it. It was so uncomfortable and agonizing.

When I pushed, I thought I was violating myself. I thought, "I can't push this hard, feeling these ripping sensations throughout my body, without hurting something."

I told the midwife, "I'm going to tear, there's no more room."
I saw her get her scissors out—she was right in front of me.
I said, "Oh, no," because that frightened me.

She said, "It will give you another inch." It did, and I didn't
even feel the small episiotomy. My fear had been unfounded.

The thing I remember, too, about the last twenty minutes, was
the eye contact between the midwife and me. She was boring her
eyes into mine, and I felt like it was just a show—she'd done it a
thousand times before. That was the face she put on when she was
in this situation. She also said these wonderful words, "With the
next push, your baby will be born." She said that about ten times,
but that's what carried me through, because I had to believe her—I
had nobody else to turn to at that point.

During the last few minutes, there was this amazing trust and
bond between us. I didn't particularly like her because she was
cheating me by saying it would happen and then it didn't.

Then my baby was born. It's worth going through it just to
experience the relief when the baby finally comes out. It must be
like being reprieved from a death sentence. It was a wonderful kind
of relief. That was it, I had done it.

I remember looking down at this purple bundle. She was bigger
than I thought she would be. I looked down at my tummy and saw
this deflated balloon—she took up more room in there than I
would have guessed.

The contractions stopped just like that. I thought of the amazing efficiency of the body and I became caught up in that. I didn't
cry. I had seen other births and so had my husband. He didn't see
our baby being born since I was sitting on his lap.

The first thing he said was, "I don't feel very well," because
there was a lot of blood. That really shocked him because he wasn't
expecting it. Actually no one prepared us. I think my midwife was
worried I might be hemorrhaging because there was so much blood.
But I was fine. That seemed to resolve itself in a few minutes.

Then she tended to our baby. Amy was kind of congested. She
had to be suctioned out a bit. That took another five or ten minutes.
They were waiting for the placenta to come out. Twenty minutes
passed and I didn't have any more contractions, which made them
a little anxious. Within minutes she told me to push a little and
then the placenta came out.

My mother was downstairs during the birth. I had invited her to be with us, but she chose not to be in the room. After they cleaned things up she came in, and I could see she'd been crying while I gave birth. It was a difficult thing for her to hear me in pain.

My attitude was, "I'm fine. I'm on top of everything." I actually took a shower and washed my hair within the hour. I wanted to do that and it felt so good.

I had lost a lot of blood and was light-headed. The midwife said, "Don't leave her alone or let her walk down stairs for twenty-four hours." Amy nursed within a half-hour of the birth. If I have another baby, I will nurse immediately. I don't see why I had to wait. If we use the birth center staff for our second baby, we'll go over what happened and revise plans for the next birth.

I had worried about being very small because I'm just under five feet. I wondered whether I'd be big enough to deliver a baby. They asked me what size my feet are, saying there's sometimes a correlation between foot size and pelvic size. Knowing that I had quite average-size feet made it okay for me to give birth at home. Obviously, if they had any doubts about my having a home birth, they would have told me. Fortunately, Amy was not a big baby. She weighed six pounds, fifteen ounces.

Introduction to Chapter 18

Two Home Births—Unplanned and Planned

Many couples decide to have a home birth, but there are important factors to consider. Women must be carefully screened, have excellent prenatal care, and verify that emergency back-up attendants and equipment are available. Please see "Introduction to Chapter 17," for advantages of a home birth.

Here are elements which rule out home birth:

1) Abnormal presentation of the baby—breech, transverse, or other abnormal position which might require last-minute obstetric procedures not possible at home.

2) Active herpes simplex virus—can be transmitted to the baby if the mother has lesions at the time of delivery. If so, a cesarean section is needed.

3) Bleeding—with or without pain, before labor, can indicate "placenta previa"(the placenta is covering the cervix and will be delivered before the baby). A cesarean section is required.

4) Cephalo-pelvic disproportion—if the baby's head is diagnosed as too large for the woman's pelvis, confirmed with a sonogram. With CPD, labor will not progress after a certain point, and a C-section needs to be performed.

5) Complications in previous pregnancies—includes anything listed above, as well as previous caesareans or a history of small-for-date babies (who have a higher risk of respiratory distress, low blood sugar levels, greater heat loss, and cerebral edema). Complications have a tendency to recur in subsequent pregnancies.

6) Diabetes

7) Women who have had six or more pregnancies have a higher incidence of uterine inertia—the uterus stops contracting.

8) Hydramnios—too much amniotic fluid.

9) Hypertension—high blood pressure, one of the unpredictable complications of birth. Have prenatal exams every week as you near the due date, and give up plans for home birth if blood pressure rises.

167

10) *Malnutrition—involves risks for the mother in labor, and may mean a small-for-date baby. Be sure to eat a healthy diet and avoid harmful substances such as alcohol, caffeine, nicotine, and other non-prescribed drugs.*

11) *Maternal-anemia—determined by blood tests. Possible effects are low birth weight and prematurity, as well as postpartum hemorrhage.*

12) *Multiple pregnancy—increases the chances of: a) small-for-date babies who require special care; b) abnormal presentation of one or more of the babies; c) separation of the placenta before the second baby is born.*

13) *Postmaturity—best determined by a twenty-four-hour urine test, to indicate if there is placental dysfunction (the fetus is no longer being properly nourished); determining postmaturity (past 42 weeks gestation) may be incorrect, because there could be an error in calculation of dates.*

14) *Pre-eclampsia (toxemia) or eclampsia—can be detected in prenatal exams. Signs of pre-eclampsia are: protein spilling in the urine; water retention in the hands, feet, face, and ankles; significant rise in blood pressure; and weight gain of at least five pounds in one week.*

15) *Rh blood incompatibility—If the mother is Rh-negative, and the baby is Rh-positive, the mother may develop antibodies against Rh-positive blood, during the first pregnancy. In a second or subsequent pregnancy, the mother's antibodies can be transmitted across the placenta, where they will destroy the baby's red blood cells, threatening the baby's health and life. If the mother is Rh-negative, there's a problem only if a blood test shows a rise in Rh antibodies (maternal antibody production) before delivery. Otherwise, immediately after birth, an umbilical cord blood sample is taken to determine if its an Rh-positive baby, and, if positive, the woman must get a Rhogam injection within 72 hours after the baby's birth.*

16) *Anyone not committed to home birth—if you're having a home birth simply because you don't like hospitals or doctors, want to avoid drugs, or are doing so from peer pressure, your reasons aren't strong enough to have a home birth.*

There is a powerful, growing movement in the United States for home births, where most births took place until the first quarter of the twentieth century. People choosing home birth generally believe it to be as safe as, or safer than, birth in a hospital or birth center.

Those who think that safety is assured by giving birth in a hospital have been misled. Complications can occur anywhere, even in a hospital setting.

Technical Reference: *Laurence D. Colman, M.D., specializing in Obstetrics, Gynecology, Infertility, and Endocrinology, Santa Monica, California*

Paula

Paula and her husband planned an ABC (alternative birth center) birth in a local hospital for their first baby. An unexpected quick birth at home led to a planned home birth for their second child's delivery.

With the first birth, I heard from a number of friends that the ABC Room was a nice experience, so I planned to use the hospital's alternative birth center room, but I had a very fast labor and she was born at home. My husband and I both wanted to be in a hospital because it was a first child and we didn't know what the experience was going to be like. We felt we needed that medical presence, you know, just in case.

I wanted as little medical intervention as possible. I don't have a lot of confidence in doctors on a regular basis, but in case of an emergency or childbirth I think it's important to have that back-up. I basically don't like hospitals: I don't like going to the doctor, so I wanted as little to do with that as possible. Since I had such a fast birth the first time, she was born at home. Everything went fine, and I thought I could certainly plan to have a home birth for my second child. If something happened that I had to go to the hospital, I could be admitted by using the childbirth center's hospital privileges. They have doctors who provide emergency services.

I chose a local birth center, run by midwives who assisted home births. My reason for choosing that was that I had a home birth that was wonderful. It was a good experience, and I didn't see any reason why I couldn't at least plan to have another home birth. I feel very lucky. I mean it worked out really well, especially with my son. I had a very good, short labor, and my husband felt comfortable about it because we had a home birth before. He was great, and he's not the kind of person who would ever have chosen that except we accidentally had a home birth and she was healthy and I was fine.

A friend of ours, who was our childbirth teacher, delivered our [first] baby. After calling the doctor three or four times, and then an ambulance, my husband finally called her and she rushed over and delivered our daughter. She'd never delivered a baby on her own, so it was as exciting for her as it was for us.

Throughout the pregnancy, I had the normal anxiety about, "Is my baby going to be healthy?" I had a lot of fears. First of all, I was nervous that I'd have a C-section because I had a bad pregnancy. I was pretty miserable through the whole pregnancy. I had a lot of aches and pains, and the last three weeks I was throwing-up every day. I realized I couldn't drink milk anymore in this pregnancy, and I eventually discovered I had a milk allergy, but I didn't know it through most of the pregnancy. I was tired and nauseous through most of the time. I felt so bad that I prepared myself for the worst possible scenario, because I couldn't believe I could feel bad during the pregnancy and then have a fantastic birth experience. I read about cesarean section, and I was prepared for that. I didn't want to have it, but I felt it was a real possibility.

I read the book Bradley wrote, *Husband Coached Childbirth,* and I definitely expected pain, but I also felt confident that I could deal with it. I wasn't freaked out by it. I felt if I had a "normal" delivery, I could handle it. Maybe that came from my mother telling me she had three unmedicated childbirths. And I felt, "I can probably do that." I talked to people who had various experiences with pain, but I felt I could get through it. I have a pretty good tolerance for pain. We took Bradley classes, I read *Husband-Coached Childbirth* and I practiced the abdominal breathing as we were taught in the classes.

I expected it to hurt. I expected to yell, even though I prepared myself to do all this deep, relaxing breathing and everything. I expected, with my first child especially, that I would be yelling, and I did. So it pretty much satisfied my expectations.

The yelling didn't bother me. I felt like, "Gosh, if you can't shout when you're in the most excruciating pain you've ever felt—when you're giving birth to a child, then life isn't very fair."

My first labor was only about an hour and forty-five minutes.

It was painful, and I yelled. I screamed at the top of my lungs at one point. I woke up and I was in transition, that's what happened to me. So it was painful, but it was fast.

I guess the yelling did release some tension.

After I had the baby, I realized I had mild contractions for about a week before I went into labor. That also happened with this baby, but the labor was different.

What surprised me most about the first birth was how fast it was and how rapidly I progressed. What surprised me the most about the second wasn't how quick the labor was—an hour—I thought I might have a short labor the second time. What surprised me was how painful it was to give birth to him. When he came out it was very painful. I didn't remember that from having my daughter. I was in pain while I was having contractions and in transition, and when she was coming down the birth canal. But then, when I was lying on the bed and she was crowning, it really wasn't that painful. She almost slid out. Whereas this baby hurt when he came out. He was a pound larger too, but I couldn't remember that intense pain from the first birth.

I could lie on my side when she was born.... Then with this baby, I was sitting up in bed with my legs spread open, 'cause the midwife had just examined me and I was dilated about nine-and-a-half centimeters or something, and I didn't want to go anywhere. I was having contractions and then he just came right through. But the sensation of his head when he was crowning was so intense [that] I'll never forget it. It was very painful. That was the only point in the second labor when I felt I had to let some noise out. Otherwise, I was much more controlled. Even though it was more painful, it's interesting, I was able to do my breathing.

The other thing was that my husband was on the phone in the first labor. He wasn't right with me because things were happening so quickly. This time he just called the midwife and that was it; he was with me the whole time. He was very helpful in keeping me slowly breathing through every contraction, which I hadn't been able to do with my daughter because it was an emergency.

My husband was either looking at me or standing right next to me, and sometimes all he'd do was [take] a slow breath himself that I'd hear, and it was enough for me so that I wouldn't make short, quick inhalations. I'd breathe slowly myself. It was very helpful. I think that had a lot to do with my ability to go through the labor without freaking out.

I think the most positive aspect of both births was the fact that I had healthy children. That's the ultimate thing. That's your goal ... to have a healthy baby. Nothing can compare with having a baby, and then when you see the baby, [and] the baby's got all his fingers and toes and is healthy. I feel lucky that I had quick births that were uncomplicated, but I would give anything to have a healthy baby. So if I had to have a C-section and be in the hospital for a week in order to have a healthy baby, fine. I think most mothers feel that way. The most important thing is to have a healthy child, and that you're healthy as well.

The only thing that was negative about the first birth was my disappointment in not being able to use the ABC room, because I was counting on it. I was all prepared, we had toured the hospital and everything. I was also disappointed that there was no one to really assist us. We had our childbirth teacher who delivered her, but she had two small children, and had to leave after an hour.

Then my husband and I were left [all alone] with this brand new baby. ... That was overwhelming. In fact, we called another friend and she came over right away. We felt like, "What do we do? Here we are, here's this brand new baby, and we don't know the first thing about it."

The nurses in the hospital would have showed us how to burp a baby, how to hold the baby, how to diaper it, help with breastfeeding and everything else.

There I was, forty-five minutes after having my baby, [and] I was completely alone. That was hard; that was real hard. So this birth I planned to have friends with me, even though I had already nursed a baby and everything. I wanted to have support from other women. That was important to me.

Unfortunately, this is the disappointing thing in his birth, the people we planned to have with us were not around when we wanted them. It was the night before Easter and a couple of our church friends were in church. There was a special service on Easter Eve. And my dearest friend, who I wanted to be with my six-year-old daughter, had gone to a lecture. So all the people we planned to [have] come to our house, we couldn't get. It turned out all right because another friend was home.... She came and basically took over with my daughter, which was real nice.

I'm thankful my husband was at home when I was ready to give birth the first time. He got on the phone and called the doctor because when I had my first real strong contraction, I couldn't call anybody. I was out of it, in transition. I was lying on the bathroom floor, totally confused. I couldn't have done anything. I would have had that baby lying on the bathroom floor, all by myself, if he hadn't been there. And the woman who delivered her, the childbirth teacher, made it a good experience for us instead of a scary experience. When she got there, she was very calming and seemed very relaxed, even though I know ... [now that] she was nervous. She helped me feel relaxed.

She came into the house, and came right to see me. I was lying on the bed and was so happy to see her. Somebody was there who knew something about this. She embraced me and saw the baby's head was crowning, but my water hadn't broken. She said, "Your water hasn't broken. Take it easy, how are you feeling?"

I said, "I really feel okay."

Then she broke the water right away, and said, "Okay, just ease the baby out. Breathe calmly and naturally, and just ease the baby out." Her voice was very calm, very soothing. She didn't sound at all nervous or worried.

Afterward, she said that when babies come out quickly there's usually no problem.

I tore just a tiny bit. My husband had called the doctor, and the doctor kept telling us to come to the hospital. I just couldn't come to the hospital. I was too far along. When the doctor came and examined me, he said I had a little tear but it wasn't worth trying to stitch. It mended quickly, and I didn't have any trouble with that.

The birth attendants for my son were wonderful from the very day I met them. There are two midwives at the childbirth center, and I liked them both. The one who delivered him was the one my husband and I met, and my daughter seemed to like her very much. She was wonderful! I knew if she was with me for my second home birth, I would be very pleased with it, and she was great. She was very relaxed. She knew exactly what she was doing. I felt completely at ease having her there. I knew she had delivered thousands of babies.

I mentioned ... before about what my husband did that was really significant. He was the most important person there, even more than the midwife, because he helped me focus on my body and the way I was feeling, and helped me breathe through all the contractions.

What I learned from my birthing experiences was [that] the best laid plans often go astray. That was definitely what I learned from both experiences. It just doesn't turn out the way we want it to. No matter what you do, it's not going to be exactly as you planned it.

What I personally gained from the experience of childbirth is knowing that I can deliver a child—experiencing excruciating pain, ... living through it, and ... telling about it. The connection with other mothers is really nice—knowing what giving birth is all about. Just having that experience is really important to me. I think it connects me to all life, no matter what fashion. It connects me to the process of life. I feel that both experiences were, though very physical, also very spiritual. So I was in awe of the miracle of having a child, and very thankful. I feel closer to God, and just closer to all life. I think having a child is the nicest thing that can happen to anybody. So I'm thankful, and that influenced my life.

Before I had children, I was more concerned with my own material possessions or my own welfare. Having children brings you outside of yourself and gives you something more important to be concerned with than your own needs all the time. It gives me a feeling of gratitude for what I have in my life that I didn't have before. If I didn't have children, I think I'd be more focused on things I don't have. When I had children I could say, "I have two great kids. I have everything."

Just last week we brought our baby to this restaurant, and we met a couple who were pregnant with their first child. They're an older couple—he's maybe fifty, and she looks like she's in her early forties. She was telling me how she really feels she's ready to give herself to something more than herself and her own life. You know she's ready to commit herself to something else.

And I said to her, "I think you have the perfect attitude for having a baby, because that's what it really takes."

I guess that's what I'd say to people. Are you ready to give up being concerned with your own universe? Are you ready to make sacrifices? Not that that's the primary objective—to make a sacrifice—but I think you have to be ready to give up some things.

175

You have to reach a point where you say, "There's more to life than just my own little life. That life should have more meaning for me than my own possessions and my own lifestyle."

When we were planning for the second birth, I was hoping to have my daughter there. We talked to her ... [and] tried to prepare her, but we always left the option up to her.

She was six, so we felt that she'd understand what was happening. [Although] she could understand the idea of childbirth, I was a little apprehensive about whether I would be shouting like I had when I gave birth to her. I was a little nervous about how she would respond to that. And I always emphasized that she had the option of going somewhere. I told my daughter, "Our friend, Nicky, will take you anywhere you want to go. If you want to go outside or to her house, if you want to go to your grandmother's house, if you want to go to a movie, anyplace."

When I went into labor, we asked her if she wanted to go to grandmother's house, since we couldn't get Nicky, after all. She said, "No." She didn't want to do that, so we got another friend to come and stay.

Our daughter wasn't really focused on me though, until right at the end, when I got on the bed and the midwife examined me. Then she came in on her own and stood at the foot of the bed. Ten or fifteen minutes later her brother was born, and she had watched the whole thing. She seemed very non-plussed about it.

She was excited after he was born. She wanted to touch him and hold him. But while in labor, I vaguely remember seeing her at the foot of the bed. I knew she was being taken care of, so I could relax about that. My friend Robin was watching Lauren, who was watching me, and she said Lauren seemed very calm through all of it. I asked her afterward if she felt frightened by any aspect of it and she said, "No, because I knew what was going to happen."

She had seen a video of a woman giving birth at home with her other children around her. And I borrowed a book from my midwife; an excellent book written for children who are going to witness birth—with lots of very descriptive pictures.... So Lauren knew what was going to happen, and it happened just the way she read about it.

I think it was a positive experience for her. I don't know what her attitude toward him would be if she hadn't been at the birth.

She is very sweet to the baby, very affectionate and considerate of him. She doesn't have any anger directed toward him at all. I would say, especially the first couple weeks, she resented that I couldn't spend any time with her, but she's never taken it out on him. She directed her anger right at me, which is who she should direct it to. So I hope the experience of her witnessing the birth will bond them to each other.

I feel the spiritual aspect of giving birth is really important, and having faith was, for me at least, the most important thing in getting through my pregnancies and giving birth—the belief that everything would be okay. I prayed quite a bit about that—either praying to God or having a spiritual connection with the rest of the world that ultimately everything would be all right. Having a good childbirth experience helps you to let go of the desire to control what's happening to you, just let it unfold the way it's supposed to. That's also something I learned from my childbirth—you can't control everything. Especially in childbirth, you realize it's not going to be the way you want it, and the best thing for you to do is relax and let it go. Release that urge to control and manipulate, and then it can be a good experience.

In the total birth experience, it's not a control thing of course. Whatever's going to happen, I have to accept that. As far as being able to get through the painful aspects without shrieking, I felt I had to do that because my daughter was there. I was working, I was conscious of the fact my daughter was there and I didn't want to frighten her. It was different when I had my daughter. I didn't have other children around, so it didn't matter.

Having my daughter at the birth motivated me to not lose my cool. My husband's presence gave me the ability to do that. He was really supportive and right with me the entire time. If he hadn't been, even if my daughter was there, I would have probably screamed, because it was very painful. So I was trying to control it, but I wasn't able to control it without him.

He was right with me for every single contraction. And it was so important for me, it was very . . . indescribable. It was just so reassuring and comforting to have him there.

Introduction to Chapter 19

Water Birth at Home

The following story discusses a woman's second home birth, with the additional element of being in warm water for labor and delivery. She decided to have a water birth, primarily for the benefit of her baby. Her intention was to create a gentle transition for the baby coming from the womb into the world, and she felt a water birth would facilitate that.

For those who want to have a home water birth, it's important to have some help in setting up the tub that is being used. In the following story, the woman used a Samadhi isolation tank, which she moved into her bedroom. This structure is shaped like a bathtub, but more square—six feet long, three feet wide, and three-and-a-half feet deep, and made of fiberglas. It was filled with about two-and-a-half feet of water, so the water reached up to the woman's shoulders when lying down.

It's suggested that the tub be set up ahead of time, by using a hose attached to a sink. The water temperature needs to be the same as the mother's internal body temperature; about 101 degrees fahrenheit. The temperature needs to be hot enough for a woman to feel the benefits, but not so hot that it might force her to leave the tub. Someone experienced in setting up the tub for a water birth would be helpful to the woman/couple planning this type of birth. The room should be heated between 75 and 80 degrees, so the laboring woman can feel warm when she's in or out of the tub.

There are inflatable plastic tubs which can be rented or purchased for a water birth. The proper assistant or assistants needed may have to be researched, since there are few medical professionals who could be hired to help at a home water birth. Lay midwives and childbirth educators who have attended many births at home are two possibilities for those who choose this type of birth.

It takes careful planning, a strong, positive attitude, and a reliable support system when attempting a home birth in general, and the same is true for a water birth in a home setting. Other suggestions are reading and becoming more knowledgeable about water births, and perhaps attending a seminar about it.

*Please refer to the Bibliography for a list of resources. There is a video called "Water Baby" by Karil Daniels, and a book entitled, **The Water Baby Information Book**, also by Daniels. Both are available from Point of View Productions, 2477 Folsom St., San Francisco, CA 94110. The phone number is (415) 821-0435.*

Technical Reference: *Pre- & Peri-Natal Psychology News, Volume II, Issue I, Spring, 1988, Steven Raymond, Editor*

Blair

Blair is a pioneer of water birthing, approximately the tenth woman in the United States to give birth this way. She used water birth at home for her second daughter's entrance to our world. During her second pregnancy, her experience with re-birthing brought up unresolved issues of her own birth, and gave her new insights into childbirth.

There are differences between a first and a second pregnancy, at least in my case. I didn't think too much about being pregnant when it was my second pregnancy, because I was so busy taking care of my first kid. There were her activities and my schedule to contend with, and that made the pregnancy less important. The first pregnancy is "the pregnancy," in my book. When it's your first, you read all the books and become educated.

During the second pregnancy, I was involved with rebirthing, which was a great thing to do when I was pregnant. I was able to get in touch with myself and learn how to be a better person. Also, it was a good time to be with others and not feel alone when I was going through my divorce. I think rebirthing is a good way for a woman to get in touch with how her own birth was, and how that can affect the way she gives birth to her baby. If you understand the impact of your own birth, that will clear up a lot of issues for the birth of your child. Then you can go through a pregnancy without the same fears that your mother had about giving birth to you. If you can recognize those fears, you don't have to repeat them when you give birth. You may still have some fears, but you won't have them on a gut level.

Although I continued receiving prenatal care from a birth center, I enjoyed floating in an isolation tank while I was pregnant. The people at the tank center were also involved in water birth. They introduced me to the idea and, after completing my one underwater rebirthing session, I experienced what a baby feels like as it's born, and knew the best way to give birth would be in water. I used a mask and breathed through a snorkel for an hour. Once I learned how to change my breathing pattern with the snorkel, I became comfortable underwater—it felt so free and safe.

During that rebirthing session, I focused on the baby I was carrying—thinking about how I was in water and my baby was floating inside me in water. While my thoughts were concentrated on my baby, I had a strong sense I was carrying a girl. I tried to think of a name for her that sounded like something to do with water.

Then my mind went to the water itself. I never wanted to come up—I was so content. I liked the temperature, and it was relaxing to be there not worrying about a thing. I felt totally safe and had my eyes closed the entire time. When I went swimming as a young girl, I often wished I could dive into the water and stay there and float, and not have to come up for air. I still wished that.

After my hour was over, I had to come out of the water. When I lifted my head and tried to take my first breath of air, I felt total panic. It was as if I didn't know how to breathe. I really didn't know what to do ... people, and lights, and air, and reality coming down and blasting me. That's it, I thought. That's what it's like for a baby being born. The baby has come from a safe, warm environment, and has a passive, yet receptive frame of mind. Suddenly, the baby's forced to breathe the air, feel the cold, hear the sounds, and be hit by it all at once.

I then understood how difficult it is for a baby to be born in the usual way. If a baby could be born in water, when she's still relaxed and feeling safe, it may make a difference for her. It would be a gentle transition from being in the womb. The temperature is different, too, because it's warmer than being in a room, out of the water. There doesn't have to be the blast of sound and air, which is so traumatic and shocking to a newborn baby.

I had decided on a home birth for my second baby, because the first was born that way and it was comfortable and easy. Now I knew I had to have an underwater birth—at home—for my second child.

My husband moved out when I was about four months pregnant with our second child, and we were going through a divorce. To replace one husband, it took five close women friends to support me during labor and delivery. If he ... [had] been there, I may have had only one woman, or two. I wanted the birth filmed, so I also had a cameraman there. A friend, who was a lay midwife, assisted me at the birth. I couldn't get a certifed nurse midwife to come to the birth, because I was doing an underwater birth. The midwife I used for my first birth wouldn't have anything to do with an underwater birth, since that was her birth center's policy.

My daughter stayed under the water about two or three minutes after she was born. When babies are born, as long as they are still attached to the umbilical cord, they are getting oxygen, so she didn't have to come up right away. Also, newborns have an inborn reflex not to breathe until they're exposed to the air. She was fine, and I think it was a nice transition for her to come into the water first, before coming into contact with the air.

When she first came out, into the water, the women let me decide when I wanted to bring her up. I watched her as she unfolded. One eye opened and then the other eye opened. As soon as both eyes were open, I lifted her just above the water and held her. She was just looking around, and I was concentrating on keeping her warm.

Amy didn't have to be forced to breathe so suddenly, since she came into the water first. Whereas, in my first daughter's— Vanessa's— birth at home, she didn't have the water experience.

If any of the psychological theories are true about the birth experience, then Amy will certainly benefit from hers. She avoided having a traumatic birth like so many people, and won't have to overcome it through something like rebirthing. One of the premises of rebirthing is that we create personal laws about ourselves, based on our experiences at birth. If you have less stuff to deal with at birth, you'll be closer to reaching your full potential. You'll have more access to being who you are without having a lot of junk to deal with.

I don't know what Amy would be like if she hadn't been born that way. She has always been a light[hearted], responsive child, who is witty, smart, and creative. I would choose underwater birth if I were going to have another baby—there's no reason not to.

I used an uncovered Samadhi isolation tank, which was moved into my bedroom ... the water reached up to my shoulders when I was lying down.

It would have been nice if the tub could have been prepared ahead of time, instead of during my labor. And I wish the water would have been kept warmer so I could have stayed in longer each time I went in.

The labor ... was okay. I stayed in the water just for short periods of time, because it wasn't warm enough. I kept getting in and out, and that was nice. It really helped to be in water for pushing. The water lifted me up in a better position than if I had been on a bed, and the water helped me go with the contractions, since I could feel my body more in the water.

The first time you go through something, you've never been there before and you don't know what to expect—it's an unknown. The second time, you know what it's like to be stuck in the process of labor, and yet I wondered what it was going to be like this time. I was a little anxious about how it was going to go. I felt closer to reality than I was during the first birth. I think that's true for a lot of women. When you've given birth at least once, there's a part of you that doesn't want to go through it again, and another part that wonders what it will be like this time. It's a task, whether it's painful or not—you have to get through it.

I don't think giving birth under water is necessarily an easier type of birth. It was very intense—more so than the first birth. My water broke and the contractions started, bam! They were hard right away and I didn't have much time to get on top of my breathing. Breathing is what makes a labor easy. If you're concentrating well, you don't feel the contractions. With my first, Vanessa, I didn't feel them. I was breathing so well because I had so many days to do it, with mild contractions that gradually built up over time. They were five minutes apart, and then three minutes apart, like a textbook kind of labor.

During the second birth, I was distracted by having more people around me. My four-year-old coming in and out of the room took away from my concentration. It takes total concentration to breathe during labor. I was more aware of the physical dimension of labor during the second birth, because I was more distracted. I was also hard on myself, because what was going on around me affected me. Inside my head, I kept telling myself I wasn't breathing right.

One negative thing that happened, during this birth, was when they cut Amy's cord too soon. It seemed to be the first time she felt discomfort, and she gave the beginnings of a cry like, "Uh, uh." I think it was too soon for it to have been cut, especially because it was still pulsing. It seemed everybody lost sight of that one part of the childbirth process. In hospitals, they don't usually wait until the cord stops pulsing to cut it.... I think [it] would be better [to wait]. It's not a big enough concern. I've seen some doctors wait, and others do it as quickly as possible. However, it was cut ... because I was getting cold and didn't want to stay in the water any longer.

Then I started having contractions, because I hadn't delivered the placenta. The midwife also wanted me out of the tub when I delivered it, so she could make sure it was all there. When Amy was three years old, I asked if she remembered her birth. She said, "Yeah, I remember. Everyone was there and I tried not to cry." That was all she said, and I thought it was really weird because what she said was true. Everyone was there and she tried not to cry when they cut the cord.

I've never asked Vanessa if she remembers her birth, and I wish I ... [had]. It's too late now, because when they're two-and-a-half to three-and-a-half years old, that's the time they have recall of it. I asked if she remembers what it was like to be at Amy's birth. Vanessa remembers me telling her to leave the room, and she wasn't happy about that. She also said she was in the tub when I pushed, but she wasn't really in the tub, she was outside of it. Vanessa did come into the tub for a little while before I was ready to push, but she thinks she was in it when Amy was born.

When Vanessa heard me crying during part of my labor with Amy, she became worried, and I asked her to leave the room. I didn't want her to see me crying and I had to stand up because I wasn't able to find a comfortable position. I told the people around me, "Please take her out." They did, and she cried in another part of the house, scared that something was going wrong. It's hard to understand a four-year-old's fears and relieve them, and the people who were helping me were worried about doing "the right thing." They didn't want me to be mad at them, so they did what they thought I wanted.

Then Vanessa noticed me being happy after Amy was born and said, "You're really happy." I thought that was a strange comment for a four-year-old to make. I expected her to say, "I'm so happy," or "We're so happy." She has always been concerned if I'm not happy.

As it turned out, Vanessa had awakened in the middle of the night, around one or two o'clock. She came in to find me in active labor—the energy of it drew her to me. The hard part was when she was with me on the bed. She'd shake the bed just a little bit, and it would break my concentration. She was trying to be helpful by giving me cool washcloths. Even at four, she was very mothering.

When the umbilical cord was cut, she saw blood spurting from it and said I told her there wasn't any blood at a birth. There really isn't, unless there's an episiotomy or a tear. Vanessa kept saying, "I know there's going to be blood when the baby's born." Then when the cord was cut, she said, "See, I told you there was blood." I think it was great that she was there. As far as her view of childbirth, I think she knows that it's painful and it takes work, but you get a baby in the end. It's a part of life, just like birth and death are part of a continuum.

It's important to find out what you'd be comfortable with, in terms of how you want to give birth. When I deal with people, especially as a childbirth instructor, I'm not a crusader like I used to be. I don't sell underwater birth, for example, or tell someone what particular kind of birth a woman should have. I'd support whatever a woman wants to have. If she wants an epidural, and I think she doesn't need one, I might tell her it doesn't seem to be necessary.... [But] if she insists on having it, I'll support her decision. I don't think anesthesia is necessary, in most cases, if a woman has a good attitude, a good support system, and if she believes she's safe during the process.

I tell women, "Childbirth is the most incredible thing you'll ever experience. When it happens, you won't believe it's normal." I tell this to every couple who comes to me for childbirth classes. I say this to them because I can't think of a better way to prepare them for what they're going to go through. If you believe you'll be safe [from the beginning of your] pregnancy, and continue that thought through labor and delivery, you'll be able to allow your body to do the work it needs to do.

I think you can feel safe wherever you are, whether you're giving birth at home, in a birthing center, in a hospital, in a car, or in a field. If women can trust the process, then they don't have to be in a hospital. They have to feel safe in their bodies, and then they'll be safe in any environment.

Whatever complications occur will happen wherever she happens to be. I think there's usually time to get to a hospital when there's an emergency. Every time I've been in hospitals, I've seen that there was plenty of time for the woman to get there from home, [and] to receive the required treatment within the time needed.

I hope I can help people have a positive birth experience, with the information I share with them. It's important to trust the birthing process, and that's difficult for many women to do. So many women don't want to trust it, or to deal with it. They just want to get someone to take care of them. Often that means being in a hospital and taking pain killers or anesthetics. They feel safe because there are people who will take care of them, and that takes away their own power. That's sad, because I think you should take charge of your childbirth experience. When a woman goes into labor, it's like being in a vacuum and you're not connected to this planet anymore. You need to have a root to keep you grounded to this world.

I chose to have women at my birth whom I felt close to. I still missed not having a man at my birth, even though I had five women assisting me. I usually didn't miss him at home—I was independent, and felt I didn't need him. So I was as surprised as anyone when these feelings of loss came up for me during the birth. They distracted me from concentrating on the birth, but once I realized I had these feelings, I talked to one of the women about them. When I made the connection in my mind and then said the words, the feelings dissipated—I didn't need them anymore.

When I'm a childbirth coach, I tell women, "If you've got something on your mind, get it out. Say it, whatever it is. If there are some thoughts you keep having, and they interfere with your breathing, bring them out—voice them, and the thought will go away."

With my second birth, I learned it wasn't necessary to have so many people around me—having two people may be enough for me. If I have more children, it is in their best interest for me to bring them into the world in a gentle way. You don't have much control over the kind of personality your child will have, but birth is one thing you have some choices about.

Part V

MULTIPLE BIRTHS

Introduction to Chapter 20
Cesarean Twins At Thirty-Nine

The incidence of twins is one in eighty-five births. If you're between thirty-five and forty years of age, and this is your first pregnancy, the chances of having twins is one in seventy-four. The use of infertility drugs increases the chances for multiple birth. Seventy percent of the time, if there is more than one baby that discovery will be made in the sixth month, using diagnostic ultrasound. Some of the signs of a multiple pregnancy are: increased weight gain, even when a woman is careful how she eats; the uterus expanding more rapidly than normal; picking up two heartbeats with a stethoscope.

Some of the problems for a woman with a multiple pregnancy are: breathlessness, varicose veins, hemorrhoids, insomnia, swelling of the legs, morning sickness, increased weight gain, and anemia.

A woman carrying more than one baby is considered a high-risk patient, and she should plan to have the babies in a hospital, preferably with the neonatal intensive care unit (NICU), should they require immediate care. Delivering twins may be easier than delivering a single child. Twins are generally smaller, and their combined weight in utero helps to open the cervix even before labor begins. One of the risks with multiple pregnancies is having premature babies. Most doctors recommend bed rest during the last trimester. They also recommend abstaining from intercourse, since that could cause the cervix to dilate prematurely and bring on labor.

Most twins are born three to four weeks early. It's safer to avoid the use of anesthetics if possible, because twins are usually so small that their respiratory systems are easily depressed by drugs.

After the birth of the first twin, the doctor waits four to fifteen minutes to see if the second twin will be born spontaneously. If the second baby does not come out after twenty minutes, the doctor usually extracts the baby. With a sonogram (ultrasound picture), the position of the twins can be determined before the birth. If both are in a breech position, a C-section will be performed.

Technical Reference: *Laurence D. Colman, M.D., specializing in Obstetrics, Gynecology, Infertility, and Endocrinology, Santa Monica, California*

Martha

Martha was thirty-nine, with three daughters, when she found out she was carrying twins. Her scheduled cesarean birth was the least of the problems she'd face as a mother of twins raising three teenage daughters.

I knew at four months [that] I'd need a C-section. There was nothing I was worried about because my third child was an emergency section. I had gone through ... labor, and then had to have a section. That was very traumatic.... This time I knew everything would be timely. I'd check into the hospital Sunday afternoon, and they would be taking the twins at eight o'clock the next morning. What scared me was the idea I was carrying two, and I couldn't think there would be two perfect babies coming out. I thought I'd either lose one or lose two. I was very concerned about their well-being.

Looking back, I wish I'd been involved with the Twins Club through the pregnancy, but I thought, "You join Twins Club after you've had twins." I didn't know anyone with twins, and there was no one for me to talk to, so that was a very lonely time. Now I'd say, if there's anyone who's going to have twins, get in touch with someone from Twins Club ... [during] the pregnancy.... There are hundreds out there who've gone through pregnancies [carrying twins] and the babies have been fine, but I was scared.

Even after three other childbirths, the fact that they were twins was hard for me.... I was extremely big and didn't feel well. It was not a pleasant pregnancy.

My first birth was nineteen years earlier, and at that time there weren't many choices. It was a quick labor; everything went beautifully. My husband wasn't involved.... I had my second daughter, fifteen months later and again there were no choices, but those were easy deliveries.

The third one was a problem. That really blew my mind! I was three weeks overdue and I was exhausted much of the time, but then I had two toddlers, too. I kept having false labor, and when I finally went into the hospital, I was six or seven centimeters dilated. Things started happening fast. The nurse checked me, and she didn't say a thing. She just put an oxygen mask on me and monitored me.

No one would tell me anything. My doctor wasn't on call that night, so they sent in another doctor who said he was watching things.

Meanwhile, they let my husband in, who was absolutely green. I asked, "What's going on?"

He said, "Oh nothing, everything's fine."

I said, "Hey, come on. I'm not a little kid. What's going on?"

Finally he said, "They're going to do a section on you if you don't deliver between now and the time your doctor comes, because the baby is in distress."

But no one had told me a thing. That was fourteen years ago, and it was very scary. I wasn't even sure what *distress* meant. As it turned out, the umbilical cord was wrapped twice around the baby's neck, cutting off needed oxygen.

I'd never had an operation before, and the "knife" worried me, too. They did the section, and then the baby was in distress. She didn't cry. Apparently the placenta had not fully developed, so that was part of the problem. The doctor said it was just a fluke. There was no reason for it, but if I hadn't been three weeks overdue, she probably wouldn't have survived because she was basically being starved. She was very small—only five pounds, and there were lots of difficulties with her.

My physical recovery was difficult, because I had bronchitis, too. I had to stifle my coughing because the incision from the surgery would hurt. I was worn out.

My mother came to help with the children for a week. When my husband had to go on a business trip, my mother offered to take the older kids to my sister's, up north, for a week. That was fine because then I had only the baby. But when she brought them back, they all came down with chicken pox. It seemed with our third child, there was one trauma after another.

Seven years later I became pregnant—quite by accident. By the time I was three months along, I looked like I was seven. I was huge. Every other week I bought larger bras. I just kept blossoming. I was tired and I didn't feel well either, but I was thirty-nine and had three kids.

When I was eighteen weeks, the doctor had me go in for an ultrasound exam, just to see how far along I was, so he could plan the section. When he said we were going to have twins, I had a fit! I started laughing because I knew if I started crying, it would be all over. I was in a state of shock!

My husband was with me, because he was very excited about this pregnancy. He was forty and having another baby; he thought it was great. And then twins—he went into orbit! He was very supportive. In fact, he's probably been more of a mother to these twins than I have. Until we had them, he'd never changed a diaper, never fed a child. Then he sort of took over. He was fabulous! He was the one that kept me going, because I was so down and not taking it well at all.

I couldn't do a whole lot of jumping around, but I was still taking care of my home and driving carpools. I became very concerned about eating—a real health nut. The part that bothered me most was that I was still smoking. I tried giving it up, and I couldn't do it. I remember a good friend said, "It's all right. You're doing enough." I felt guilty about smoking and carrying two babies, but I could only cope with so much at one time.

From the time I was four months along, I was very uncomfortable. I was so big, I couldn't sleep. I wasn't comfortable lying on my side, because all that weight was on my ribs. It was just awful! The last five months, I never had a good night's sleep. I finally had my husband buy me a hammock, and we strung it in the family room. He would help me get into it, and I'd lie on my stomach ... to relieve the pressure on the rest of my body. By October, my maternity clothes didn't fit anymore!

I just kept getting bigger and bigger and bigger, and I retained a lot of fluids. I was always hot, and waddled around. I couldn't even sit like a lady. I gained fifty pounds, and weighed 185 pounds when they were born.

After the birth of our third child, I thought nothing could ever be that traumatic. I knew I'd be in the hospital without labor pains.

There'd be no possibility of having them before I could make it to the hospital. And another thing, everybody says twins come early. The C-section was scheduled for January twenty-second, but I made up my mind on Thanksgiving that any day they'd be coming. So that last five weeks was very long, because I went right to the end. They were full-term.

I went in Sunday at two in the afternoon, and at six o'clock the next morning they started preparing me for surgery. One was born at eight o'clock and the other at eight-oh-five.

When the first one was born, the doctor told me it was a girl. I had really been hoping for one boy, maybe not two, but one. Then when they took the second one, the doctor said to my husband, "You tell her."

And Tom said, "You know it's another girl."

My next question was, "Are they okay?" And once they said, "Yes," and showed them to me, I didn't care about the sexes. They were beautiful, and I was glad to have been awake to see them.

Having a section was easier then, 'cause I always got cold and had shakes after having the other kids. There was none of that; this was much easier.

My tubes were tied right after the twins were born. When the doctor had told me I was pregnant the fourth time, I didn't even discuss the pregnancy. I said, "Hey, we're talking tying my tubes. Let's not even talk pregnancy." He kept laughing at me. I said, "No, this is a major thing and we're not going through this again!"

I guess I was a little sore from that procedure, because he had to do a lot of poking and tugging. They didn't let me get up until late that night, but I was fine.

Lorna weighed five pounds, nine ounces, and Carla weighed four pounds, eleven ounces. And that's with smoking.

Lots of mothers in the Twins Club had seven or eight pound babies. These women are big ladies to begin with. But I remember going to the Twins Club, and they said mine were small compared to most babies in the club. But I always thought they weren't small, and I know they weren't.

The most positive part of having twins was the excitement. My husband was there … the pediatrician was present. When it's twins, everybody all over the hospital peeks in and says, "Oh, it's twins!" It was like a big party. The same way when we checked in—the nurses all came around, the doctors, the anesthesiologists. There's something very special about twins. Everybody gets concerned. They all want to know what's going on.

I was real high from the birth. They were fine. My three other daughters came to see me, and I received cards from all the kids at school. I was on cloud nine. It was fun for about two-and-a-half weeks. Then reality set in when everyone went back to work: here I am with two infants.

It was very depressing, because you can't go anywhere with two. I didn't have help, so I felt trapped. And, in feeling trapped, I started feeling sorry for myself—poor me. I did a lot of crying. I felt overwhelmed. It wasn't until they were about three months old that I said to myself, "You don't have to be trapped if you don't want to be. You can put them in a stroller and you can go up the street. You can get out." And I forced myself out.

I started thinking about attending a Twins Club meeting. They were born in January, and I think the first meeting I went to was in March. Then I didn't even want to go because it was such an effort to just get up and get dressed. There was so much going on.

My favorite story is when the babies first had really messy diapers. They each had one at the same time, and I was looking at them, trying to decide which one to start with. Suddenly, my twelve-year-old came into the bedroom crying because she just started her period.

I thought, "I can't deal with this. I cannot deal with going from dirty diapers to puberty!" It was hard coping with two babies and teenagers at the same time.

My daughters helped out, but they needed me, too, and there was only one of me. My husband was very good, but with five kids and two of them infants, there was always so much work. The kids were good to help feed them. Tom did all the night feedings so I could sleep, and he looked pretty haggard.

It was hard because I couldn't go anywhere alone. I mean I couldn't even take them to the doctor without someone helping me. I'm kind of an independent person, and it was difficult for me to ask people, but I needed help. Even to go to the market for a quart of milk was a three-hour deal.

I'd say, "I can't handle these kids." I was getting depressed, and then I thought, "I can't do this to myself. If I really want to get out,

I can." I began taking the babies for a walk, and ... [I'd] see older ladies and men smile at the stroller, and it was making their day. That's what really started getting me through it—the attention. There were a lot of nice people out walking, and they'd peer in and ask, "Are they twins?" They were so happy to see these little babies that I felt, "If I can put a smile on someone else's face, it's really not so bad."

I learned a lot from having my twins. From the time I was pregnant until they were about a year old, my prayer was always, "Why me? There are so many people out there who want children and can't have them, and three is enough for me." You know, I didn't need two more really, and yet they've brought so much joy to our family. So even though I thought I knew so much, there are times when things happen without my understanding, and it's been positive for our whole family. It brought us all much closer. I've seen a different man in my husband, so it's been good.

When we were expecting our first daughter, I didn't even take Baby Care [Baby Care is a Red Cross course that gives instruction for couples about bathing, feeding, and postpartum care for the baby and mother.], because I worked until two weeks before she was born. The information we have today wasn't available then. Nineteen years ago, I wasn't that involved with my giving birth. I just remember walking into the hospital with my suitcase, having a wheelchair waiting for me, and sort of being whipped into it. They got rid of my husband, and I was in this room with them going through their routine. I was alone and didn't know what to expect. That was scary. Then, when I was going through labor, I kept thinking, "I don't want to go through this—I'm leaving! This is not what I want."

Even my mother didn't tell me what giving birth was like. She was knocked out for both her childbirths. She doesn't even remember they shaved her. She didn't know anything.

Today, my feeling is a lot of people are having children because it's one more thing they want. It's in the plan. I think when you have a child, or children, *that* is a job in itself. It's something that starts from the day you're pregnant and lasts for a lifetime. Motherhood isn't just a phase or something you're going to do. I mean, you can't get rid of this. It's there forever and it emotionally drains you. You have your highs and lows, but you can't walk away. It's a big responsibility. Your lives are going to change.

You can't think just of yourself anymore. That person is there. You're totally responsible for that person's well-being, right down the line. You don't pop this kid out and turn it over to a baby sitter or someone. People need to think about these things. Kids don't just grow up. They need your influence. They need you to be around. You don't [just] have a child.... You can't put this child away and close the door. It's not a job you're going to work at for five years and it'll be over.

What kind of adults are we raising? That scares me. Try spending as much time as you can with someone who already has a child and see what it's like. Your relationship with your husband changes too. It takes a couple years for the two of you to become a family. My husband, being an only child, had an extremely hard time sharing. He didn't talk about it, but I could see there was jealousy when the babies began to arrive.

I advise, "Think about having children. Know what you're getting into. It can be very rewarding, [but] it can also be very, very depressing."

Before I had children, I was a secretary at a corporation.... Then suddenly I was home alone with the babies. I resented my husband taking off and doing his thing, and there I was stuck in an apartment with walls all around me.

I never had time to do what I wanted. I ... [should] have quit work when I was six months pregnant—to go out for lunch with friends, do things just for me, because the minute that baby comes, you've got to get a babysitter. It was a time I should have taken and didn't. I'm still waiting for it!

Two Sets Of Vaginal Twins

In the following story, a woman was carrying a set of twins and didn't know it. Her doctor hadn't ordered a diagnostic ultrasound, even by the twenty-fifth week of pregnancy. Ten years ago, which is when this happened, doctors were more hesitant about taking a sonogram (the picture that results from the diagnostic ultrasound method). Now, they are much more common, and are recommended when twins are suspected for any reason.

Multiple births are riskier for mother and babies alike. Usually there's more weight gain, which puts more strain on the bladder and the ureter—increasing the chances of a urinary tract infection, which can lead to pre-term labor if the infection goes undetected and/or untreated. Carrying multiples is harder on a woman's body, because all the internal organs are crowded with two or more fetuses growing and taking up space.

Many twins are delivered by C-section, since they are often premature. They also tend to have a smaller birth weight, and one or both may be in a breech position. Therefore, a vaginal delivery would be too risky to attempt.

Some *doctors require a certain amount of bed rest throughout the pregnancy, to encourage a longer gestation period for the babies. And* ***most*** *doctors suggest some bed rest, especially in the last three months of pregnancy.*

*If pre-term labor is threatening to start, at the onset of contractions the mother can be given terbutaline—**in a medical setting.** Terbutaline relaxes the uterus, increases the heart rate of the mother, and has been the drug of choice to prevent pre-term labor. The safe use of terbutaline has not been definitely established. Its therapeutic benefits have to be weighed against any yet-undetermined risks to the mother and child. In both mother and baby, terbutaline increases heart rate and blood sugar, while reducing potassium. This medication should be given only when your doctor decides it's absolutely necessary. Terbutaline has the fewest side-effects of any medication used to treat pre-term labor.*

Technical References: *Laurence D. Colman, M.D., specializing in Obstetrics, Gynecology, Infertility, and Endocrinology, Santa Monica, California; Norman Goldstein, Doctor of Pharmacy, Santa Monica, California*

Amy

*Amy and her husband had two sets of twins; the first were
born at twenty-seven weeks, and the second at thirty-five
weeks. This moving story describes both the elation of becoming parents, and the heartbreaking loss of children so
desperately wanted.*

The first was a very much wanted pregnancy. My husband and
I had infertility problems for some time, but we worked that out.
We went to an infertility specialist for seven months, and eventually
used artificial insemination—plus plenty of medications—to
achieve this pregnancy.

I finally did conceive, and the pregnancy went beautifully.
Since I was seeing an infertility specialist, and because we had a
rocky start, we chose not to tell anyone—except medical people—
about the pregnancy for three months.

After the first trimester, I transferred from the clinic to an
obstetrician. I didn't know I was carrying twins, and therefore at
risk during this pregnancy. We were joyous about finally having a
baby, and let the whole world know. Monthly, I saw the obstetrician
and was treated as a low-risk patient. Retrospectively, I'm not sure
that was the best way of handling it.

There was always the chance I could have twins, because of the
medications I was taking before insemination, but I never got a
clue from any of the medical people that I was carrying more than
one baby.

Each time I visited the doctor, I'd ask, "Do you think it could
be more than one?"

And he said, "Gee, I don't think so."

I only suspected it might be more than one because of the
medications, and because we do have some twins in the family.

At one point, I was visiting the obstetrician, and my measurement was less than it had been the month before, which alarmed me. I was re-measured, and the doctor said, "Well, the baby moves around a lot." We were reassured to know the baby moved around a lot, and we thought everything was fine.

We set the next appointment for a month later, which would have been the six-month check-up. The appointment was on a Tuesday. On the Friday night before the scheduled appointment, I had a cold and wanted to get some extra sleep, so we went to bed early. At eleven o'clock, I woke up because the bed was drenched. I called my doctor and said, "I think my water has broken."

He said, "*When* are you due? This seems highly unlikely." He went through a number of questions, and said it might be a high leak in the amniotic sac, and it would seal. He thought I might have lost bladder control, and I told him there was no odor so it was definitely amniotic fluid.

He said, "I don't think it's anything to worry about. Call me if you have any additional symptoms; like bleeding, cramping, contractions. Otherwise, give me a call in the morning."

I didn't sleep very well the rest of the night. I was up and down to the bathroom, and worried. My first reaction to my husband was, "I'm not ready to have this baby." I knew it was too early and I was frightened. The doctor didn't seem concerned about it. From the point where I am now, of course, all that was very wrong, but I was naive and trusting.

About six o'clock in the morning, I was bothered with a lot of gas pains, which is something I don't ordinarily have. It finally dawned on me that what I was feeling might be labor, so I timed the gas pains ... they came in regular intervals.

It was around seven when I put all this together in my head, and ... called the doctor. The pains weren't what I thought labor should feel like—I was just a little uncomfortable. There was nothing else going on, related to what the doctor said to watch for. I called him and he wanted me to meet him in his office. I was still very trusting when I went to see him.

He examined me and said, "Yes, you're going to have a very premature baby." This doctor didn't practice at a hospital which handled premature babies, since they didn't have a neonatal intensive care unit. As a matter of fact, he did office births, and he delivered babies at a community hospital which didn't have any high-risk care.

He arranged for another doctor to handle the delivery at a large, well-equipped hospital. I just had to get to the hospital, which seemed like the other end of the world but wasn't really that far. Because of the circumstances, I simply moved, without questioning things like distance, in order to get the care I needed.

We arrived and I remember being admitted and talking to the nurses. They asked me how far along I was, and when I said I was twenty-seven weeks, they said, "No, I don't think so."

And I told them, "I know exactly how far along I am because I had artificial insemination."

Another nurse came in and said, "So, you know exactly how far along you are. Are you also equally sure you're only having one?"

And I said, "Well, no, I'm not."

The question had been raised, but nothing more was said. Everyone was congenial at that point, and I was directed into a labor room. I can remember the experience being very unreal. Everything was happening far too fast.

My husband left to make a couple of phone calls, so at least a few people and our minister would know where we were. When we left that morning, we didn't know we were going to have a baby, so we didn't want to give out too much information.... We really didn't know ourselves what was happening.

When my husband left to make the calls, I remember feeling numbed by the whole experience. I saw a very close friend come into the room, peek in, not sure she should be there. Talking to her later, she wasn't sure she should have come at all, [since I seemed unaware and unresponsive]. I wasn't really "out of it"—I was very aware she was there, but in a kind of "twilight zone."

There were people coming in and out of the room, none of whom I knew. My obstetrician, who was my one tie to this experience, wasn't going to be there. It was a teaching hospital, so residents kept coming and going. They'd try to put a monitor on, and they'd want to check me for cervical dilation.

One of the things my obstetrician said before I left his office was, "Don't let them give you an alcohol drip, because that's not good for the baby." I still hadn't met the obstetrician who was going to deliver, and I felt desperately in need of a "team captain." All I arrived knowing was I wanted the best for this baby, and not to have an alcohol drip.

Suddenly, they said they were going to give me something to stop labor. I was terribly naive and didn't know what was happening. The physician who was going to deliver my baby hadn't arrived yet.

I said, "I don't know. Is it something my doctor wants me to have?" At that point, they became defensive and angry with me because I was refusing the services they felt were necessary.... I wasn't telling them "No," I was just uncertain. They went out in a huff.

The nurses came in, looked at the monitor, ... looked at me, and said, "Oh, you're not in labor. If you were really in labor, we'd be seeing much more movement on the monitor."

That particular comment was made about thirty seconds before the physician walked in. He took one look at me and said, ""Now *that* was a good contraction. Let's get you into the delivery room, STAT." So it was really a day and night difference between how the nurses and the doctor interpreted my condition.

Jack came back from making the phone calls and was told he couldn't go into the delivery room. They said there wasn't enough room for him—he is a quadriplegic, in a wheelchair. I think they felt there wasn't time to help him get in so he could see and help with the birth.

The new doctor was there and seemed very pleasant. I had confidence in him simply because my obstetrician had referred him. On the way into the delivery room, I told him, "You know, I haven't been to any of the childbirth classes. I don't know what to expect or what to do. You're going to have to coach me all the way."

He said, "That's fine. It won't be a problem."

In the delivery room, there wasn't a need for anything, until the doctor decided an episiotomy was necessary to reduce the trauma for a premature baby. So I had a local for the episiotomy. The doctor coached me through it and I delivered the baby.

I remember the whole thing was a bit of a blur, because it was happening in such an unreal fashion. I certainly remember some discomfort, but nothing incapacitating. I remember hearing a weak, little cry and feeling elated.

No matter which sex I would have preferred—and I don't remember whether I had a strong opinion about it—it didn't make a bit of difference. I had a baby; the baby was alive, and I heard a cry. I could see down over my knees, as they were reaching and ... [passing] this tiny baby from one hand to another, it was a very red, scrawny, weak-crying baby.

I was real thrilled. They told me it was a girl. It was another piece of information, but it really didn't matter. It was a baby and she was alive. She needed immediate care because she was so small, so they couldn't bring her to me and let me touch her.

I didn't have much experience with premature babies, except for visiting a neonatal intensive care unit (NICU) as a teenager. Having worked with handicapped children who started life in incubators in a NICU, I knew there'd be lots of intervention after birth.

I'm not sure anyone told me what to expect in terms of her size. It turned out she was one-thousand grams, or two-and-a-quarter pounds. I turned to the doctor and said, "I don't know what to do next."

And he said, "Just lie there. Sometimes when there's a premature baby, the placenta won't be delivered that quickly. Let's just wait and see what happens."

It was only a matter of minutes when I said, "I feel the same thing again." From under his mask I could see a quizzical look on his face. He reached in and then came back out, and said, "Uh-huh, there's another one."

So it wasn't, "Here comes the placenta." It was, "Here comes another baby."

At some point he said, "Push," and the baby emerged. This was a little boy, and I didn't hear him cry. I didn't have a sense of impending doom, but I didn't hear him because there was so much going on in the room. They had called for another team of people, since there was another baby to deal with.

I remember the doctor holding the placenta and saying, "This is the placenta."

And I said, "That can't be, because it was a boy and a girl—there have to be two." Part of my energy was used to argue with him. I had no control over anything else.

After the second baby was born, I asked him, "How many more? Are you sure we're done?" We didn't know there were going to be two, so I wondered if there were any more babies. It took me a bit to get that one resolved.

The babies were taken to the NICU for care. My husband asked the staff what I had. When they said I had a boy and a girl, he said, "Not *my* wife!" He was so surprised I had two, and he went to see them soon after he came in and saw me.

I went back to my original obstetrician for follow-up. He said, "From seeing you that morning in the office, I would have sent you for a diagnostic ultrasound that month, because your measurement was significantly larger."

The twins died after three weeks in the hospital's NICU They were on ventilators the whole time, although our daughter was taken off for one day and put on a machine one step-down from that, which is called, "continuous positive airways pressure (C-PAP)," to wean her off the ventilator. She was on that for a day, and then had to go back on the ventilator the next day. They said she had become sick, and they gave her medications. They didn't seem to think it was significant that she had to go back on the ventilator. She died that night. The infection she had was very serious, and [it] took her quickly.

With our little boy, we knew from the time he was a week-and-a-half old [that] he had some major problems. They were doing everything they could, but nothing seemed to improve the situation.... He had a downward course for the next week-and-a-half. We became very involved with, and attached to, the NICU, and were glad it was there.

One family in particular was very supportive to us, and we were to them. Their baby was there for months, and I went back to visit that baby and the family. Part of doing that was for me, not just for them. It helped me to work through the loss—it was so abrupt to stop something which had such a huge impact on our lives. I kept going back and visiting, and we became close to a lot of people there, including the Director of Neonatology. A number of months after our babies died, another parent who had twins there, approached the director about starting a support group for the unit. The director thought about it and looked back over the records of families whose babies had been in the unit over the past few years.

Because we had maintained contact with him and the staff since our twins were born, he called us. Obviously, it wasn't because ours was a great outcome, and that was true for some of the other families he called. Many of us had become closer to the unit as a result of losing our babies. We joined the original support group for families whose babies had been in the NICU.

I think we knew, even right after they died, we'd want to attempt another pregnancy. Not to replace them, but we wanted to have children, and we'd try again.

We did some things differently for the second pregnancy. As I mentioned, my husband is disabled and I always took on most of his care. I continued to do that during this pregnancy as well, but I also brought in someone to help.

I don't think that made the difference, but I can't say for sure. I was doing a little less lifting, but I was lifting all along.... Some people gave me their lay opinion on why I had the twins so early, and they thought I was doing too much physical work.

The doctor never understood why I went into labor so early, and ... that wasn't too helpful. But, in a way, it ruled out some things. The only thing they could say was that twins are more likely to come early. That wasn't reassuring to hear when twins were confirmed at eighteen weeks into my next pregnancy.

It was almost a year from the twins' birth to when I conceived the second time. That meant, it took us six months before we started trying again.... I was back at the infertility clinic, with the same doctor, for the first three months.

I changed obstetricians, [but] not because of blaming him for the way he handled things the first time. In fact, I wouldn't allow myself to blame him or feel he did things inappropriately. Looking back on it now, I think he could have done things much better. Then, I justified changing obstetricians because I wanted to be at a hospital where emergencies could be handled, especially because my experience made it blatantly clear that if I need it, I need it now and not in two hours. I was no longer a candidate for an office birth, and I didn't want to be in a community hospital. Those settings couldn't offer a full-range of services if they were needed.

So much for a wonderful, home-like birth! The health of the mother and the babies is more important. Sure, it would be nice to have those few moments—cozy and comfortable, with low lights and quiet, and family all around. That would be an ideal, maybe. But it's … ideal [only] if you know everything can be taken care of that needs to be. For my own comfort, I needed to be in a hospital that could deal with emergencies. I knew I was at risk again, since I was taking medications that increased my chances for multiples. I now had a record of a premature birth. I was definitely a high-risk patient, so I wanted to select an obstetrician who delivered in a hospital, preferably the same hospital where I delivered my first twins.

Even though our outcome was bad, I felt tremendous about the care the babies received. I didn't always feel so positive about the experience I had as a patient, but I felt very good about what they got, and that was the bottom line, in my opinion. I thought, "That's where I want to be if I should again deliver early." I'm an optimist, and I was sure it wouldn't happen again, but I wanted to cover the bases.

I found an obstetrician by interviewing a number of them, through referrals from friends and also from the doctor who delivered the first set of twins. This doctor who had stepped in at the last moment said he'd take me on as a patient, but he thought it might cause me undue stress to travel so far. He referred me to someone closer to my home, who'd deliver at the hospital I preferred.

That was the best of all worlds—to have a doctor nearby who could admit me to the hospital I wanted. I had my first appointment with him at about seventeen weeks. He thought he'd do a diagnostic ultrasound at some point to see what we were dealing with. At this appointment, he examined me and measured the uterine growth. After he told me the measurement, I had him repeat it. He wrinkled his forehead, and thought I should have an ultrasound the next week.

The sonogram [ultrasound picture] showed twins. I had mixed reactions—tremendously joyful and excited, but apprehensive. Things had to go right this time, [and] I just knew they would. I was not going to sit around being a "basket case." It wouldn't do the babies or me any good. I knew there were risks and I knew we would do anything to lower them. There wasn't anything we did inappropriately in my first pregnancy. I didn't live with guilt about the twins' death.

I probably should have gone on bed rest when it was going to make the biggest difference, the point when I delivered the first time, at twenty-seven weeks. But I didn't, and everything was going fine, and I was very confident about my pregnancy. After that day, everything beyond was victory. I made it another day, I made it another week. And from then on, everything was just pluses. It was a wonderful way to keep going with the pregnancy. No, I didn't want to deliver at twenty-eight weeks or twenty-nine or thirty. But each one was longer than the time before. Thirty weeks isn't when you want to deliver, but past thirty the survival rate is significantly better.

Somewhere around thirty-two weeks, I came down with the flu. I was hospitalized and monitored for awhile, just to make sure it wouldn't become a fever-induced labor. I did fine, even with higher blood pressure. I was pretty sick with the flu, and survived for the next ten days on "Gatorade."

When I recovered, I had lost ten pounds and had some problems with my legs. Another doctor found I had some veins blanching down my legs, giving me some pain. They had to determine whether I had clots or what. The tests were uncomfortable.... They couldn't find anything, but wanted to redo them in two days.

The morning of the day I was to return for the second round of tests, I awakened at six, because my water broke. I was at thirty-five weeks, and that was wonderful! We knew at thirty-five weeks [that] they weren't going to stop labor in an aggressive way.

When I called the doctor that morning, I said, "Okay, my water has broken, and remember, I'm going to the larger hospital."

We went to the hospital and after he examined me, he said, "We're not going to stop labor, but we're going to buy as much time as we can. No bathroom privileges, and I want you on an IV. We're just going to do things as cautiously as we can, to buy hours of time. We can't buy weeks now, only hours."

Every additional hour the twins could be kept inside, the better chance their lungs would be developed. That's what we did, and I had another ultrasound during that day. We found out number two was a boy. We didn't know what number one was, because there was inadequate fluid around that baby to be able to see the genitals. They were both doing just fine.

209

The day nurses were very good. They were pleasant, and I was their first twin patient. They'd move the monitor belts all around my stomach, trying to get them to read, and of course it was hard to get them [to read properly] on two babies. These nurses responded to what I said, which was nice.

The [nurses' shifts] changed and, unfortunately, so did their attitudes. One nurse couldn't be bothered getting the belts right, to be picked up well by the monitor. I was now in heavy labor. With this pregnancy, I went to childbirth classes, so I knew more about what was happening....

By late afternoon, I was in active labor and asked the nurse if she had called my doctor. I felt he needed to hurry, because I thought the twins were going to be born soon.

The nurse said, "Oh, you're not that close yet." This nursing staff wouldn't listen to their patient. They had their technology. I'm the first to agree technology is extremely important, having been through the experiences I have, *but* you sure have to do more than use technology. You also have to use some common sense and listen to the patient.

They finally pulled in a resident, because they got so annoyed with me. He said, "Yeah, you're going to deliver all right." There wasn't much of a chance my doctor would ... [arrive] before delivery, but they called him and reassured me he had been called.

Another doctor stepped in and introduced himself as a friend of my obstetrician. We agreed he should deliver the twins if my doctor didn't arrive on time.

The nurses had a hard time getting the IV started on me before the delivery, so they called the anesthesiologist. He started the IV in the delivery room, and did what any one of the nurses could have done—he ... [inserted] a small needle into my hand instead of the larger one the nurses were trying to get in.

Again, I didn't need any medication, except a local for the epiosotomy. They did an ultrasound that morning to specifically determine the position of the twins. If they weren't both vertex [head-down], a C-section would have been performed.

I was tremendously grateful they were both vertex. I didn't like the idea of a C-section, nor was I mentally prepared for it. I was thrilled they could be born vaginally, because earlier in the pregnancy they were in a transverse position [lying horizontally].

For the first one, everything went smoothly. My husband was in the room, and able to coach me. I still felt like I didn't have it all together from the childbirth classes—I was denied practicing in the different positions, as a precautionary measure. Some of the nurses helped me with the positions, since my husband couldn't physically help me.

I pushed the first one out—a little girl, and healthy. My husband and I were absolutely thrilled at that moment, because we not only had what looked like a healthy baby girl, we knew number two was a boy. So we had a boy and a girl again! In no way was that a comparison or a replacement for the first two. It was just wonderful to have one of each sex. We were ecstatic!

After she was born, the doctor wanted to rupture the membranes on number two and put a monitor on. I said, "Why, for heaven's sake? Everything looks like it's going well, and you don't have any indication that there are any problems. If you don't see any reason to do it, why should we rush this? Besides, my doctor's on the way, and maybe he'll get here for the second one." That sounded novel to him, I guess, and he didn't have a good retort for it.

As it turned out, my obstetrician was not on the way, but I still didn't want this doctor to rupture the membranes and hurry things along. It was the weekend replacement doctor who was coming, because it was now Friday evening. It was not only Friday evening, but my doctor had an emergency in his office that no one told me about.

I was disappointed that my doctor couldn't be there, however, I had met the back-up doctor during the pregnancy. They felt it was important for me to meet him, in case my doctor couldn't be at the birth. He was perfectly fine, but it wasn't like having the person I was hoping for.

It was a half-hour between the two births. I again had a cold before I went into labor, but somehow my body had its priorities straight, and said, "Forget this! Cold goes on hold, we're delivering babies now." I was fine through the whole delivery. I didn't have any signs of a cold. That was an interesting dynamic I watched my body undergo.

We had this half-hour waiting period when we were able to lie there and be happy about what was going on. We had a healthy, beautiful, little girl. I saw her before they took her to the nursery. She weighed five pounds, and a half-ounce.

Thirty minutes went by, and then I honestly can't remember the details. Probably I started contracting again. Right before I began to push, everyone thought it was going to go smoothly. After all, I just delivered a baby! I thought everything was open and the baby should slip right out. Wrong! This kid had a bigger head, and wasn't coming out easily at all. I pushed with great effort, and a very bruised head emerged—he was fine. He was taken away to be measured and weighed—he was even bigger—five pounds, nine ounces. Things went well, and it was just a matter of stitching me up and transferring me to the recovery room.

While in recovery, they brought the babies in, which really pleased me. When they brought in our son, he wasn't breathing too well—we kept wishing our pediatrician would hurry up and arrive. The baby was not in terrible distress, or they would have rushed him upstairs to NICU. Overall, they were doing well.

It was a couple more hours before the pediatrician came and examined the twins. When he told us our son needed to go to the NICU, we didn't panic. A lot of people who have heard our story think we would have been alarmed by that, since we had been through it once before. The reason it didn't bother us … [was that] there was such a big difference between the two sets of twins. He was not a tiny, sick baby, but a good-sized baby who needed some help.

Our daughter never went to NICU, although she stayed in the hospital beyond my discharge. She was jaundiced and had to stay under the bili lights for six days.

> *When a baby has jaundice, it means there is a higher than necessary level of bilirubin—a by-product of hemoglobin—in the blood. The fetus requires a high level of bilirubin in order to obtain sufficient oxygen from the placenta, but after the baby is born it doesn't need the same level, since there is now air to breathe. If the liver doesn't break down enough of the bilirubin, the bili lights will. The baby is usually placed under the lights for six hours at a time, and then off for six hours, until the bilirubin is reduced to a normal level.*

> **—Laurence D. Colman, M.D.,** Santa Monica, California

They called us when she reached the normal level, which meant she could be taken home. We went at ten o'clock at night to pick her up. They said we had to bring her back the next morning, so they could test her again. We didn't care—we were taking a baby home! We were able to spend a few hours with her that night, and it was wonderful!

When we brought her back to the hospital the next morning, we visited her brother upstairs. He had mild preemie problems—he needed oxygen, some blood, some feeding encouragement, and he had to learn to keep his temperature up. He did those things pretty quickly, and came home three days after his sister.

Even though it was a twin birth, they were two distinct deliveries, half-an-hour apart. They each had their own separate time and experience. And our son and daughter have been different all along, ... but very close to each other. However, everything about them has been individual—their temperaments, feeding styles, their abilities to deal with the world around them.

When I knew I was at risk for twins, but didn't know I was having twins in the first pregnancy, I remember saying, "I hope it's not twins, because I won't be able to give each of them the time and involvement I would like." I really wanted to focus on one baby. Of course, I had misgivings after saying that and then having two. I desperately wanted them both to live, but they didn't. And I did ... want them.

The second time, I was of course thrilled, because we had missed the chance of raising twins. Here we were given another chance to parent two children at once. An interesting thing about having twins the second time, is that I wasn't surprised by having twins, yet our infertility doctor was. I thought the doctor, of all people, shouldn't have been surprised. I suppose he thought he had it so well-controlled that it wouldn't happen again.

I have some biases with regard to what to tell a woman who's expecting twins. They're based on my own experiences, as well as from my professional viewpoint, since I have worked in the NICU for four years. Of course, not all mothers of twins are going to have premature babies, but the babies are at an increased risk—particularly for prematurity. More often, it is more like my second experience;... weeks early, rather than months.

If the doctor recommends cutting down on activity, or being confined to bed rest, or anything, even though these things may not be proven they may give your babies a better chance. The long-term goal of ending up with healthy babies has to be the priority. It may inconvenience people, and it may not be the ideal pregnancy they envisioned, but I feel strongly that why you go into a pregnancy is to end up with a baby—a baby you can raise, that becomes part of your life and part of society. And that goal is still there, and really has to take precedence over momentary conveniences for the mother. We were lucky when we were going through the experience with the first set of twins. Our family and friends were very supportive, but many people have a different experience. I now work part-time as a support person with new parents, in connection with the social workers and the staff of the NICU, to help meet some of the needs of the new families. It's more than just a tiny baby we're treating when there's a fragile baby—it's a whole family.

Looking back on our first experience, I was eager to go meet my babies, and it took hours to finally see them, since they had taken me away from them, out of the postpartum unit. Then they had to transport me quite a distance—from the surgical wing to the NICU. I couldn't walk there—it was against their policy. My out-of-town relatives were able to see my babies before I did. That was aggravating—I felt cheated.

A lot of mothers don't want to be in the postpartum unit. They don't want to be hearing other babies or seeing babies taken into rooms—surrounded by everyone excited about a healthy baby they're going to take home. So some mothers prefer going to the surgical floor.

There was a lot of denial of motherhood by doing that, and I think there really is a middle ground. One way would be to offer the mom a choice. But if you can't, and the system is to have her go to the surgical floor, there should be an explanation and the staff could be more supportive. They should also tell her that visitors can come in and out more easily on the surgical floor, and that can be very important when a new mom is separated from her baby.

However, I was ... [warmly] welcomed by the NICU. The moment I got there, [while I was still] outside the door [and] hadn't even gone in or been told where to scrub yet,... a nurse said, "Oh,

214

this must be the mother of the twins." She was so warm and wonderful, and told me what was going on.

Since I had small babies and a fairly easy delivery, I wanted to get out of the hospital as fast as I could. My babies were there, and I wanted to be near them, but I couldn't even get transportation to get to where they were. I checked out the next morning, put my things in the car, and then went up to see my kids. Then I could visit them as an out-patient—as a mother instead of as a patient, and it worked much better.

The term "bonding" is probably ... [overused] or it's ... [used] in such a way that it seems restrictive in the ways it must happen; ... this magical thing called "bonding." It isn't that you have to have your baby on your breast two minutes after he exits the body—that isn't what bonding is all about. You can have a tremendously close relationship with a baby who's very sick and very fragile, although it doesn't happen for everyone. I bonded to my first set of twins even though they were taken away so quickly. The fact that I couldn't get to see them within the first few hours didn't interfere with my ability to bond with them. That's why I'm working with the NICU, because I was very close to it. If I hadn't made an attachment to those babies, I wouldn't have made such a close connection to the staff and to the hospital.

During the [second] pregnancy, I was bonded to the fact that there were two, but I never really knew this kid on the right or that one on the left [although] I've talked to mothers of twins who knew one twin from the other when they were pregnant.

We have photographs of our first twins [that were made] during the three weeks of their lives. These pictures are so important to me. We found out when we shared the photographs with people while the babies were still alive, that some people could handle seeing them and some couldn't. Some of the pictures weren't that scary to look at, considering some of the stuff hooked up to them.

If you didn't have anything else in the picture, people would say, "They don't look so small." But if one of us placed our hand in the picture with them, they looked very tiny. The pictures were extremely important to me after they died. That was part of my ... [coming to terms] with their death. One of my great fears was I'd forget what they looked like. The pictures made it more concrete for me.

We didn't take pictures of them after they died. It wasn't suggested to us, but it fleetingly went through my mind—and seemed bizarre. At the time, there are things you're afraid to deal with, and you think they look strange.

I'm a real advocate of it today; I do it for people all the time. I take photographs and videos for families at the hospital, of their premature babies when they're alive, and also when they die. No one has said, "Don't do that." Once they have the pictures, parents can choose to look at them later. They can't look at them in the future if they were never taken.

It's true that twins bring an increase in work and exhaustion, but there is also an increase in rewards. To be able to enjoy them and learn as much as possible about each of them as an individual, and not just as a pair, is really important. It's a very special thing to have twins.

In Closing

The women who shared their personal birthing stories for *Childbirth Choices In Mothers' Words* are greatly appreciated for their candor, sensitivity, and openness. I was surprised how easily they talked about their diverse adventures, and the lasting impact made on each woman's life.

It's not my intention to make judgments or to recommend one particular birth method. Many books tell you what they think is the healthiest, easiest, or the most natural way to give birth. This book is different because the women's words are the most important part.

My part was just to "get the facts" and inform readers of the diversity of birthing experiences. I hope these stories serve as tools to educate and enlighten women about the total picture of birth, not to present a narrow view about a particular method of birthing.

There is something within this book for all women. The reader needs to make her own choices about what will work best for her pregnancy and childbirth. Women who have already given birth will make their own discoveries about their birthing experiences. They can compare and contrast these stories against their own or other women's experiences, and perhaps gain some fresh insights. Others may pick up some new information which might change the way they have a future baby.

My own birthing experience was a difficult one, but it taught me valuable things. Because of the kind of birth I had, I learned how important it is to prepare for the unknown. If women have fears well in advance of the birth, they should seek out help, so they can prevent unnecessary intervention during birth. Fear has a way of repeating itself during the birth process, when apprehension has not been dealt with beforehand.

It is helpful for women to try and anticipate what's most likely to occur when they give birth, and to balance that with what they'd most like to have happen. It's also important for them to visualize the kind of birth they'd like to have, and for them to believe they can create it.

Women shouldn't be afraid to admit they're scared. Experiencing birth can be the most frightening experience in one's life especially when women don't feel reassured and comforted during their pregnancy and subsequent birth.

Having support during birth is the most important factor for a positive birth. You'll hear it over and over again from women who've said they couldn't have gone through the birth without having someone there with them. That person can be her husband, friend, sister, mother, anyone, as long as she feels supported by them.

I hope *Childbirth Choices in Mothers' Words* will be used as a valuable resource before, during, and after pregnancy, even if it has been many years since your child was born. If this book is used simply to learn more about the female experience of birth, I will be glad I wrote it. If readers gain deeper insights into their own birthing experiences, I'll feel greatly rewarded by my efforts.

I hope you have benefited from reading my book. I'd appreciate any comments you have.

Kim Selbert

Bibliography

Ashford, Janet Isaacs, ed. *Birth Stories—The Experience Remembered.* Crossing Press, 1984.

Berkow, Robert, ed. *Merck Manual of Diagnosis and Therapy, 15th Edition,* Merck & Co., Inc., 1987.

Berman, Salee, C.N.M. and Victor Berman, M.D. *The Birth Center—An Approach to the Birth Experience.* Prentice Hall, 1986.

Burck, Frances Wells. *Mothers Talking—Sharing The Secret.* St. Martin's Press, 1986.

Chamberlain, David, Ph.D. *Babies Remember Birth.* Tarcher, 1988.

Cohen, Nancy Wainer and Lois J. Estner. *Silent Knife—Cesarean Prevention & Vaginal Birth After Cesarean.* Bergin & Garvey, 1983.

Friedland, Ronnie and Carol Kort, eds. *The Mothers' Book—Shared Experiences.* Houghton Mifflin Company, 1981.

Greene, Bob. *Good Morning, Merry Sunshine.* Penguin Books, 1985.

Israeloff, Roberta. *Coming To Terms.* Knopf, 1984.

Jones, Carl. *Visualizations for an Easier Childbirth.* Meadowbrook, 1988; and *After the Baby Is Born.* Dodd, Mead, 1986..

Kitzinger, Sheila. *Your Baby, Your Way—Making Pregancy Decisions & Birth Plans.* Pantheon, 1987.

La Leche League International. *The Womanly Art of Breastfeeding.* La Leche League International, 1981.

Leboyer, Frederick. *Birth Without Violence.* Knopf, 1975.

Markowitz, Elysa and Howard Brainen. *Baby Dance—A Comprehensive Guide to Prenatal and Postpartum Exercise.* Prentice Hall, 1980.

Marzollo, Jean. *9 Months, 1 Day, 1 Year—A Guide To Pregnancy, Birth, and Babycare.* Harper & Row, 1975.

Mayer, Rochelle, Ed.D. *Beginning Together—A Diary Of Discovery For You And Your Baby.* St. Martin's Press, 1983.

Noble, Elizabeth. *Childbirth With Insight.* Houghton Mifflin Company, 1983.

Odent, Michael, M.D. *Birth Reborn.* Pantheon, 1980.

Rakowitz, Elly and Gloria S. Rubin. *Living With Your New Baby—A Postpartum Guide For Mothers And Fathers.* Franklin Watts, 1978.

Richards, Lynn Baptista. *The Vaginal Birth After Cesarean Experience.* Bergin & Garvey, 1987.

Spacek, Tim. *Fathers—There At The Birth.* Chicago Review Press, 1985.

Star, Rima Beth. *The Healing Power Of Birth.* Star Publishing, 1986.

Stukane, Eileen. *The Dream Worlds Of Pregnancy.* Quill, 1985.

Sussman, John R., M.D. and B. Blake Levitt. *Before You Conceive—The Complete Pregnancy Guide.* Bantam, 1989.

Verny, Thomas, M.D. with John Kelly. *The Secret Life Of The Unborn Child.* Summit Books, 1981.

INDEX

Other Books Available From Mills and Sanderson

Thirteen National Parks with Room to Roam, by Ruthe and Walt Wolverton. Discover those under-utilized parks that lack the pressing crowds but have the beauty, charm, and facilities you want. $9.95

The World Up Close: A Cyclist's Adventures on Five Continents, by Kameel B. Nasr. Discover the essence of humanity through various cultures by vicariously wandering the world by bicycle. $9.95

The Alaska Traveler: Year 'Round Vacation Adventures for Everyone, by Steven C. Levi. With maps and cartoons, this is a unique insider's guide to gold panning, stalking big game, windsurfing, dogsledding, etc. $9.95

The Portugal Traveler: Great Sights and Hidden Treasures, by Barbara Radcliffe Rogers and Stillman Rogers. A companion to fascinating places to eat and sleep, festivals and other events as well as insider tips to enrich your visit. Includes city maps. $9.95

Sicilian Walks: Exploring the History and Culture of the Two Sicilies, by William J. Bonville. Self-guided tours (with maps)of Sicily and the adjacent Italian mainland. $9.95

Bedtime Teaching Tales for Kids: A Parent's Storybook, by Gary Ludvigson, Ph. D. Eighteen engrossing stories to help children 5-11 work through problems such as fear of failure, sibling rivalry, bullies, divorce, death, child abuse, handicaps,etc. $9.95

Your Food-Allergic Child: A Parent's Guide, by Janet E. Meizel. How to shop and cook for children with allergies, plus nutrient and chemical reference charts of common foods, medications, and grocery brands. $9.95

Winning Tactics for Women Over Forty: How to Take Charge of Your Life and Have Fun Doing It, by Anne De Sola Cardoza and Mavis B. Sutton. For women left alone through separation, divorce or death, "this title presents many positive, concrete options for change." - *The Midwest Book Review* $9.95

Fifty and Fired: How to Prepare for It - What to Do When It Happens, by Ed Brandt with Leonard Corwen. How to deal with getting forcefully "restructured" out of your job at the wrong time in your career. $9.95 /$16.95 (hardcover)

Aquacises: Restoring and Maintaining Mobility with Water Excrcises, by Miriam Study Giles. Despite age, obesity or physical handicaps, anyone can improve their fitness with this instructive illustrated handbook. $9.95

60-Second Shiatzu: How to Energize, Erase Pain, and Conquer Tension in One Minute, by Eva Shaw. A helpfully illustrated, quick-results introduction to do-it-yourself acupressure. $7.95

Your Astrological Guide to Fitness, by Eva Shaw. Ideal exercises, sports, menus, and related gifts for those born under each sign of the zodiac. $9.95

Bachelor in the Kitchen: Beyond Bologna and Cheese, by Gordon Haskett with Wendy Haskett. Fast and easy ways to make delectable meals, snacks, drinks from easily obtainable ingredients. $7.95

Order Form

If you are unable to find our books in your local bookstore, you may order them directly from us. Please enclose check or money order for amount of purchase and add $1.00 per book handling charge.

( ) Levi / *The Alaska Traveler* $9.95 _____
( ) Rogers / *The Portugal Traveler* $9.95 _____
( ) Bonville / *Sicilian Walks* $9.95 _____
( ) Ludvigson / *Bedtime Teaching Tales for Kids* $9.95 _____
( ) Wolverton / *Thirteen National Parks with Room* $9.95 _____
( ) Meizel / *Your Food-Allergic Child* $9.95 _____
( ) Nasr / *The World Up Close* $9.95 _____
( ) Cardoza/Sutton / *Winning Tactics for Women* $9.95 _____
( ) Brandt/Corwen / *Fifty and Fired* $16.95 (cloth) _____
( ) Brandt/Corwen / *Fifty and Fired* $9.95 (paper) _____
( ) Giles / *Aquacises* $9.95 _____
( ) Shaw / *60-Second Shiatzu* $7.95 _____
( ) Shaw / *Your Astrological Guide to Fitness* $9.95 _____
( ) Haskett / *Bachelor in the Kitchen* $7.95 _____

$1.00 per book handling charge _____
5% sales tax for MA residents _____

Total amount enclosed _____

Name: _____

Address: _____

City: _____ State: _____ Zip code: _____

Mail to: Mills & Sanderson, Publishers
442 Marrett Road, Suite 6
Lexington, MA 02173
617-861-0992

Our Toll-Free Order # is 1-800-441-6224